THE DALES VET

A Working Life in Pictures

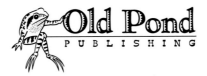
Old Pond
PUBLISHING

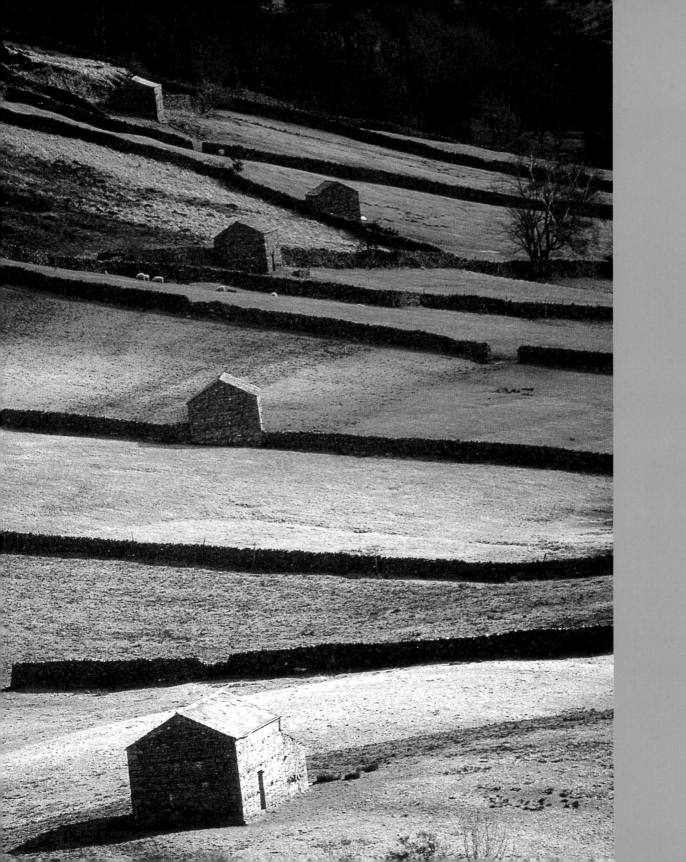

THE DALES VET

A Working Life in Pictures

NEVILLE TURNER

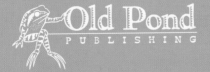

First published 2016

Copyright © Neville Turner 2016

Published by
Old Pond Publishing

An imprint of 5M Publishing Ltd,
Benchmark House,
8 Smithy Wood Drive,
Sheffield, S35 1QN, UK
Tel: +44 (0) 0114 246 4799
www.oldpond.com

A catalogue record for this book is available from the British Library

ISBN 978-1-910456-51-4

Book layout by
Keystroke, Neville Lodge, Wolverhampton

Printed by
Replika Press Pvt Ltd, India

Photos by Neville Turner

Contents

Acknowledgements

Ian Findlay MBE and Dr Margaret Bradshaw MBE, two friends with encyclopaedic knowledge of the natural history of the dale, for generously sharing their knowledge with me.

The Hill Farmers of Teesdale for adding to my understanding of the landscape and culture of the dale.

Everyone at Dalesman Publishing who have supported my work for many years.

Stewart Bonney, editor of The Northumbrian, for his encouragement by publishing much of my early countryside writing in his magazines.

Polly Pullar, fellow writer and animal-lover, for her friendship.

Rachel Turner, commissioning editor at Old Pond Publishing for her enthusiasm for this project from day one.

To my wife Chris.

With love and thanks.

Introduction

Books by veterinary surgeons are legion, and it's flattering to know that our working lives have been of interest to generations of readers. There are stirring tales of derring-do, and stories to bring a tear to the eye. Good though many of these books are, there's none to touch the master of the genre, Alf Wight, the creator of the wonderful James Herriot stories.

"The Dales Vet" does not pretend to follow in his footsteps.

There are, it's true, lots of veterinary anecdotes scattered among the pages, but in putting this book together, I set out to do something different. I wanted to paint a picture of the joy of being a rural vet in a very special landscape.

In my busy working life in Teesdale I reckon that I drove about 35,000 miles each year for over 30 years. A little mental arithmetic reveals that I travelled over a million miles in the High Pennines, which is equivalent to driving to the moon and back twice. As you can imagine, that gave me an abundance of wonderful opportunities to gain an intimacy and deep knowledge of all aspects of this gem of the English countryside.

It also gave me an abundance of opportunities to make a photographic record.

In my travels there was always a camera within reach, and it only took a few seconds to stop and take a picture. The resulting collection of images runs into the tens of thousands. It documents my

working life, the life of the hill farmer, the awesome
landscape, the culture of the dales, and my passion
for natural history.

This, I believe, is a unique picture collection, and
I am indebted to my publishers for presenting a
part of it to a wider audience both within the dale
and beyond.

1 The Best Job in the World

I recently came across a folder in the bottom of my filing cabinet containing my junior school end-of-year reports from 1952 to 1955. At the bottom of each is space for the form-teacher's comments on interests and aptitudes. The 1952 entry runs, "Interested in all subjects—especially nature study and outdoor subjects". In 1953 it was "Takes a keen and intelligent interest in nature study". The following year, "Takes a keen interest generally, but especially nature study". And in 1955, "Keenly interested in nature study".

Clearly, by the tender age of eight I had become not only aware of, but fascinated by the beauty and wondrous order of the natural world. The interest never faded. In fact it has stayed with me, deepened, and played an important part in my life.

It seemed a logical step to follow a career that would be challenging, rewarding, interesting, and give me the opportunity to keep in touch with nature. The life of a veterinary surgeon in rural practice was tailor-made to my requirements, but to spend thirty years of my working life travelling in the fantastic landscape of the Pennine Dales was a bonus. Each working day provided an opportunity to observe the ever-changing face of this unique environment day by day, season to season, and indeed over an appreciable span of years. I feel so privileged to have gained such an intimacy with the natural history and the people of the dales.

It was a funny old life being a vet in a large country practice forty years ago. If it had been a normal nine-to five-job it would have been quite civilised.

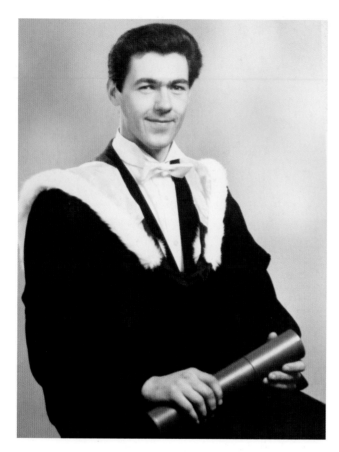

Graduation, 1968.

However, nights and weekends on duty, early starts, and late finishes made for a strange lifestyle. Not having the luxury of shift work, a night on duty was sandwiched between two very demanding working days, and a quiet telephone between six pm and eight-thirty am was a rare occurrence. It's only recently I've realised that for fifteen years the pattern of my working life consisted of thirty-six hours on duty followed by twelve hours off duty. And a working weekend stretched from Friday morning to Monday evening: four days and three nights non-stop.

As I hauled myself out of bed in the middle of the night to attend a calving, I'd mutter under my breath, "This is a savage way to make a living," but once on the road I'd be full of youthful enthusiasm, anticipating the impending case.

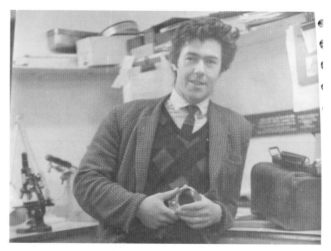

Rural practice in the late 1960s was just like the world of James Herriot.

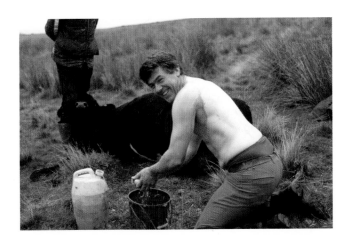

Attending a case on the moor. Miles from anywhere, but lots of hot water, a bucket, and a new bar of soap were on hand thanks to a thoughtful farmer. However, they always forgot to bring a towel!

Little more than ninety minutes later my colleague and I were drinking a welcome cup of coffee back at the surgery, having successfully dealt with the lot! We were extremely tired, but we glowed with a warm feeling of job satisfaction.

Demanding it may have been, but there were bonuses over and above the job-satisfaction factor.

Every day during the quieter spells in summer I was travelling at a leisurely pace through some of the most beautiful countryside in Britain. There was time to lean on a dry-stone wall and soak up the tranquillity and beauty. There was time to gain an intimate knowledge of the natural history of the

I well remember a Saturday evening several years ago during a particularly busy spring. My colleague and I had each been on the road for thirteen hours without a meal-stop. It was nine pm. I'd completed all my calls and stopped the car to radio to base. I couldn't believe it. There were two of us on duty and the crackling voice on the radio announced that there were five emergency calls to deal with—two ewes lambing, a cow calving, a dog injured in a traffic accident, and a cow blowing up like a balloon because of a potato stuck in its throat.

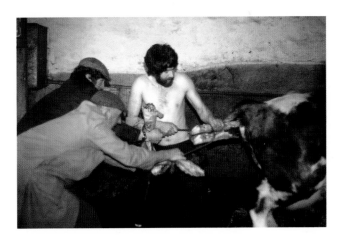

Calvings were always dramatic.

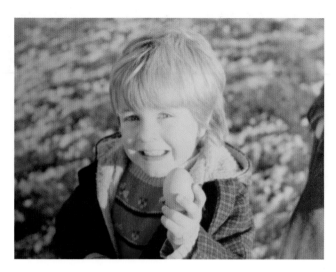

Dan collects eggs on one of my farm visits. Dan calved his first cow when he was three years old.

toddler stage through to starting school, and again in school holidays I could count on their company. And what fun we had. There's an old saying that the most precious gift one can give to one's children is "time", and I was in a unique position to do just that.

Arthur and Daniel would enjoy exploring, playing hide-and-seek in the hayshed, making the acquaintance of puppies and kittens, and watching me work with cattle, sheep, and horses. The boys soon learned, too, where to expect a kindly farmer's wife to appear with a glass of milk and some biscuits.

dale. There was time to strike up deep friendships with the dales farmer, a character whose wisdom, knowledge, talents, and sense of humour were second to none. On a good day it was like earning my living by visiting friends.

And there was another bonus.

Many fathers leave for work before their children go off to school, and arrive home just in time for bath time and a bedtime story. However, for many years I had the joy of having one or both of my young sons with me on working days. From

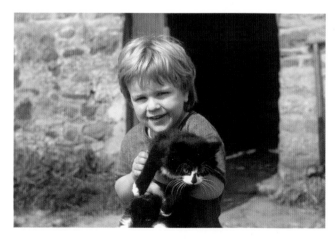

Dan gives a reluctant farmyard kitten a cuddle.

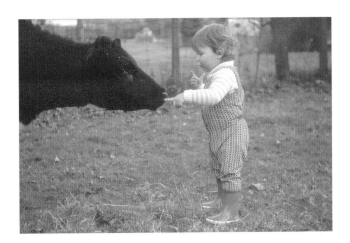

Arthur announces that this is the calf's nose.

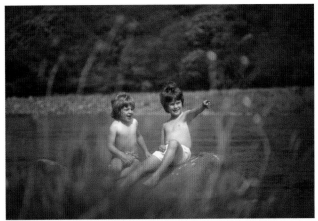

The boys take a break by the Tees.

Experiencing the miracle of birth was always exciting, and the boys enjoyed calls to calvings and lambings. On one occasion, at the tender age of three, Daniel "assisted" at his first calving.

I had completed my initial internal examination of the cow and all was well. This was going to be straightforward. The calf was alive, and presenting itself in textbook fashion with head tucked neatly between two extended forelegs. There was plenty of room in the dam's pelvis, but the exertions of labour had made her simply run out of steam. The calf still lay well inside the cow, and was going to stay there unless we intervened.

The procedure in this case is quite simple. The birth canal is lubricated, and a rope is attached to the calf's head and to each of the feet. Vigorous traction on each of the ropes, in synchrony with the cow's weakening contractions, will complete the operation.

However, before the farmer and I started the big heave, I handed one of the leg ropes to Daniel and asked him to pull as hard as he could. Reaching inside the cow, I gripped the relevant leg and eased it forward. As a calf's foot came into view on the end of his rope, Daniel's face was a picture. He was calving a cow!

The farmer, enjoying the moment as much as I was, gave me a knowing wink, and added to the fun by presenting Dan with a shiny 10p piece for "helping to calve my cow".

Eddie Straiton, famous as the "TV Vet" in the 1970s, once had a letter published in the *Veterinary Record*, in which he said,

// Despite the bad old times of seven day weeks and up to twenty hours a day with only the odd short break and modest financial reward, most of my generation would, I am certain, still describe their dedicated lives as holidays with pay. How very fortunate we were, and still are, to be members of the best of professions. //

I'll second that.

2 The Old Order Changeth

"The old order changeth, yielding place to new," wrote Tennyson.

Sixties graduates are very fortunate in that they caught a glimpse of what I affectionately and very respectfully refer to as the "James Herriot era". Flair and initiative, crucial in any profession, were even more important than they are today. One flew by the seat of one's pants, albeit armed with a wealth of knowledge and skills accrued during the gruelling five-year course.

The flamboyant characters in the wonderful books by Herriot (Alf Wight) were not just figments of a fertile imagination and a prolific pen. They were everywhere. There were dozens of real-life Siegfrieds, Tristans, Jameses, and even Granville Bennetts. Whilst I never met any of the actual individuals on whom these characters were based, I was privileged to count scores of similarly colourful characters as my friends and colleagues.

"'Tis an imprecise art which we practise," ran a quote in the final-year magazine, published for our graduation. Progress would render those words increasingly invalid. We sixties graduates were to witness an astonishing revolution which would equip our profession for the high-tech twenty-first century.

An armoury of new drugs was discovered. Machines could process blood samples in minutes, to give accurate results for haematology and biochemistry. X-ray and ultrasound scanning devices became part of the normal equipment in general practice. Research identified diseases that had not been previously recognised or treated. While individual clinical cases were still an integral part of our daily workload, preventive medicine became more important, controlling disease by management and vaccination programmes.

"The old order" certainly saw many changes.

When I joined the practice in the early seventies, it was manned by four vets. We operated out of two rooms, each about twelve feet square, rented from the gas and central heating engineer next door. Total practice assets comprised a desk, a chair, a telephone, a filing cabinet, a safe, a table, and four cars that had seen better days.

The atmosphere was positively Dickensian, but it was a happy and busy practice, typical of most dales practices at that time. Household pets did not play an important part in our workload, since the premises could not accommodate anything but the most minor surgical procedures.

In the late seventies the opportunity arose to rent a two-up/two-down house just up the street, and we seized the opportunity. The front room became the office, doubling as a waiting room, while the back

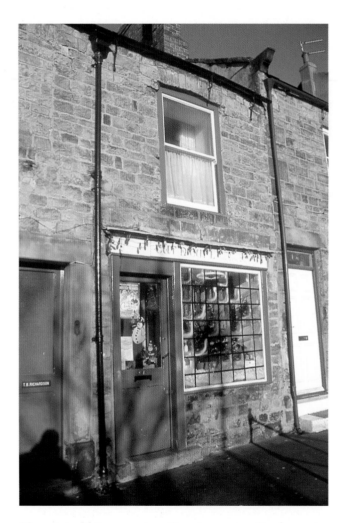

The original bijou premises. Two tiny rooms. Total practice assets were a desk, a chair, a telephone, a table, a filing cabinet, a safe, and four secondhand cars that had seen better days.

room became a drug store, doubling as a consulting room. The two upstairs rooms were converted into accommodation for one of the assistants. It was during this phase in the firm that it became a truly mixed practice.

The extra space allowed us to take domestic pets more seriously. When the office staff left at five pm, the large front room became a waiting room for dog and cat owners. Our surgical skills developed to a point where only the most complicated cases needed referral to a larger, better-equipped practice. We purchased our very first X-ray machine, and set up a darkroom in the cellar where we could process the plates. Horse ownership was becoming more popular at this time and the equine workload became heavier.

Service to the dales farming community still occupied most of our working day. This service took a giant leap forward when our first two-way radio system was installed in the cars. No longer would we have to keep a supply of 2p coins in our pockets, and find a phone box at regular intervals during our rounds to check for emergencies. We were in constant contact with the office.

Occasionally, by chance, we would be passing a farm as the farmer made an emergency call. We

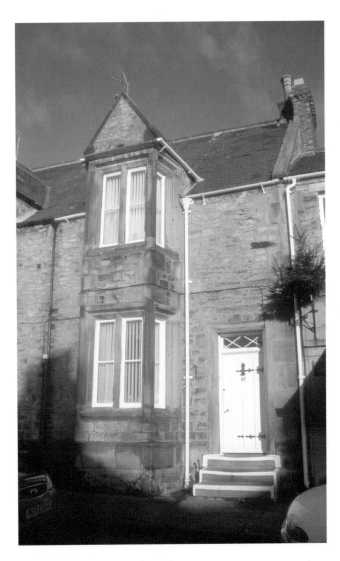

Renting a two-up, two-down house gave us some space to take small animals more seriously.

could be in his yard before he had put the phone down. I'll never forget the amazed expressions on the faces. On one occasion a client recovered from his amazement sufficiently to ask where I'd parked my helicopter!

We soon found the problem of limited space was making life difficult, and when some warehouse space fifty yards up the road came on the market, we leapt at the opportunity to own our own premises. We could design the interior to our specifications and needs.

We were thrilled at the result—lots of space, good access, and a position conveniently on the edge of the busy town centre.

Within the building we had incorporated a waiting room, two consulting rooms, a dispensary, kennels, operating theatre, preparation room, dark room, administration office, reception area, drug store, and even a large conference room. A third of the floor space was retained as a vast barn into which horses, sheep, and occasionally cattle could be brought for attention.

This was the ultimate. This was perfection. This, we fondly imagined, was where we would happily spend the rest of our working days. But we hadn't reckoned with "the old order". It was still "changeth-ing".

The most obvious change was a gradual but relentless one. It was happening in all the picturesque market towns in the eastern foothills of the Pennines. It was traffic congestion. These towns were not designed to handle thousands of motor cars passing through or parking. By the early nineties our wonderful purpose-built premises were suffering from the fact that neither we, nor our clients, could get in!

Alongside this a less obvious and even more relentless change was taking place. One has always needed to know a lot to be a competent veterinary surgeon, and to remain competent it is necessary to constantly keep up to date with new techniques and developments. I believe that at some point the state of knowledge within the profession was expanding so rapidly that it became impossible to know everything about everything. And so, in this tale of evolution, a new species evolved—the specialist.

Gradually, almost without realising it, each veterinary surgeon was showing a leaning towards one of the three disciplines that made up veterinary

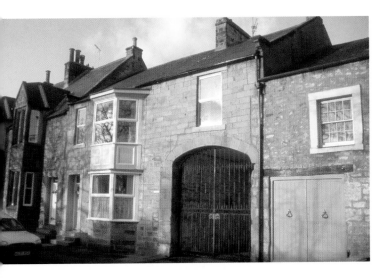

The first premises we actually owned. We converted a warehouse into purpose-built facilities. It was perfection. We could hardly imagine that we would ever outgrow it, but we did.

practice—equine, farm animal, or companion animal. It was impossible to be a "Jack of all trades" any longer. It was about this time that we heard the sad news that Alf Wight, creator of the stirring James Herriot tales, had died. I was struck by the poignant thought that, alongside him, the James Herriot-type vet had died too.

By the mid nineties we realised we would have to abandon our in-town site, and move again. Congestion in the town, and the needs for modern specialist facilities dictated this decision. Being a general practice determined to provide a comprehensive veterinary service, we needed to find a building on the outskirts of town with good access and parking, and room to create three specialist departments under one roof.

After a long search we found the ideal solution— a large empty factory on an industrial estate on the immediate outskirts of town. Again we had purchased a large (this time very large) box and had the freedom to design what was to go into it. Each of the three disciplines came to an amicable agreement on the plans and allocation of space.

In July 1997 we moved into premises that we could scarcely have imagined twenty-five years before. Here we could deal with the needs of equine, small animal, and farm patients in the same caring manner as always, but with ease of access and facilities that ensured the best of treatment.

A month later we held an open day, and entertained over two thousand visitors in three hours. The official opening ceremony was performed by Dorothy Peacock, who had joined the firm in its original bijou premises. Her retirement happened to coincide with our open day.

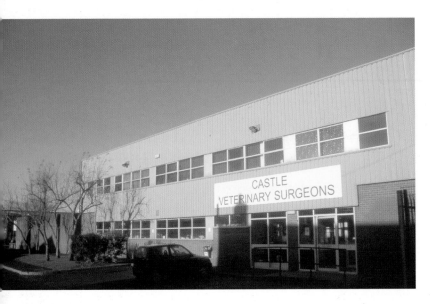

A redundant factory which we converted into a practice fit for the twenty-first century, with equine, small animal, and farm animal departments. In the new premises there were fourteen specialised veterinary surgeons and over twenty lay staff.

In the early days Dorothy, with a little part-time help, had run the office. She was receptionist, secretary, nurse, wages clerk, accounts clerk, and stock controller rolled into one. In the new premises there were fourteen vets. Over twenty lay staff were employed to carry out the functions that Dorothy performed single-handed.

If you need to know how the old order changeth, ask Dorothy. She was there and held our hands through it all.

3 A Blow for the Village

"Neville, there's a trumpet on the doorstep."

Christine had gone to bring in the milk and I was just opening the newspaper.

"A what?" I called back.

"A trumpet," came the reply.

I stopped reading the paper and went to the door to see the phenomenon for myself. There had been other unexpected objects left on the doorstep many times: the odd brace of pheasant or grouse, a sack of apples, and on one occasion a whole Stilton cheese, but never a musical instrument.

"This isn't a trumpet," I said.

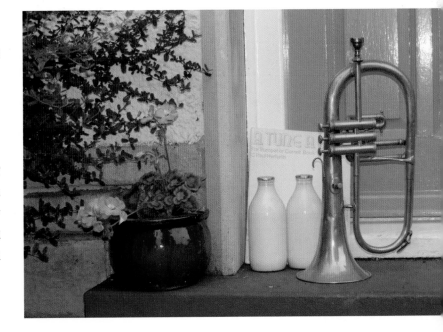

How a flugel horn arrived with the milk.

Chris looked at me as though I had taken leave of my senses.

"No, no, it's a flugel horn, a kind of trumpet," I explained.

"Yes, dear," said Chris as she took the milk to the fridge.

I picked up the instrument. All now became clear to me. A few days earlier I had been talking to Joss Allison, one of our farming clients, who was concerned that the village band was not at full

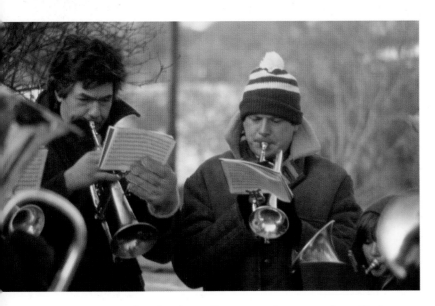

My first banding efforts were playing carols at Christmas.

strength, and was in need of some new members. He, himself, had been a member of the band for decades, and I mentioned, casually, that at school and college I had played the trombone in a traditional jazz band. In a similarly casual manner, I had mentioned that one day I might, just might, take up a brass instrument again.

I had not expected my tentative offer to join the ranks of the local ensemble at some point in the future to be taken up with such alacrity.

Mickleton is a peaceful village, and David Rabbitts knew that when he left the old flugel horn on my doorstep, it would remain safe until we took it in. He was not only our local milkman, but also the percussionist in the Middleton and Teesdale Prize Silver Band. Joss had obviously asked him to deliver the instrument in the hope that I would take the hint.

There was no note of explanation. Nor was there a phone call to ascertain my willingness to learn how to play. Such is village life.

Handling the instrument and blowing a few tentative notes reminded me of the fun to be had from music-making, and I practised for several weeks in the run-up to Christmas. What I lacked in talent was adequately compensated by enthusiasm, and

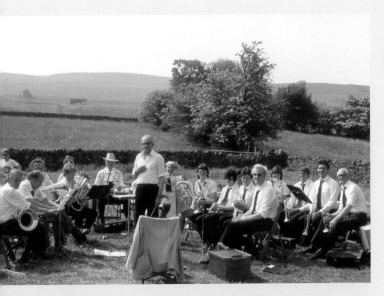

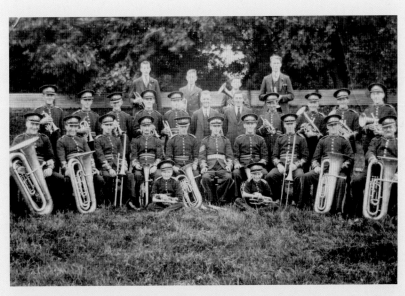

Summer concerts at village carnivals were a delight.

New uniforms in the thirties.

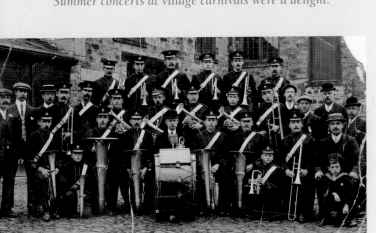

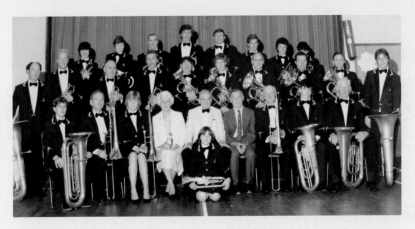

Middleton and Teesdale Prize Silver Band in new uniforms, 1910.

New uniforms 1980. I'm in the middle of the back row with a new flugel horn.

I chose to make my debut with the band on their annual evening of carol-playing around the streets of the picturesque village of Staindrop. I arrived unannounced, enveloped in my grandfather's old overcoat and a scarf of Dr Who proportions. Under convenient lamp posts we stopped and played two or three of the old favourite Christmas carols, to the obvious delight of householders, and passers-by in the chilly night.

Thomas Hardy in *Under the Greenwood Tree* immortalised a church orchestra, a body of worthy and enthusiastic amateur musicians drawn from all walks of country life. The whole of the first chapter focuses on their caroling. This, however, was Teesdale in the twentieth century, not Wessex in the 1890s. And though the dialect and scenery couldn't be more different, that December evening I felt very much a part of such an orchestra, and the band and the hearty singing of rural folk convinced me that the spirit of Thomas Hardy is alive and well, and living in our dale.

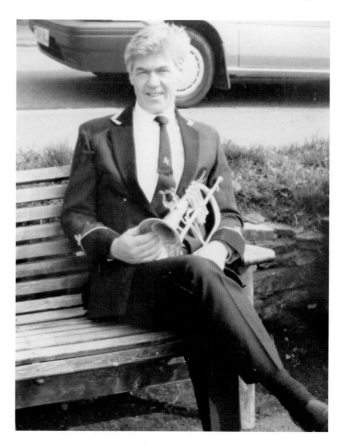

The author in uniform at Middleton carnival.

The eight o'clock Christmas Eve service is the highlight of the year for me. The church is always tightly packed with people who have left their firesides and braved the biting wind to be there. At the end of the service, when the last "amen" has been sung, and the blessing given, the ladies of the parish pass round cups of tea and mince pies while the band play a short concert of Christmas music, and end the evening with a few rousing choruses of "Jingle Bells". To emerge from the church to see a

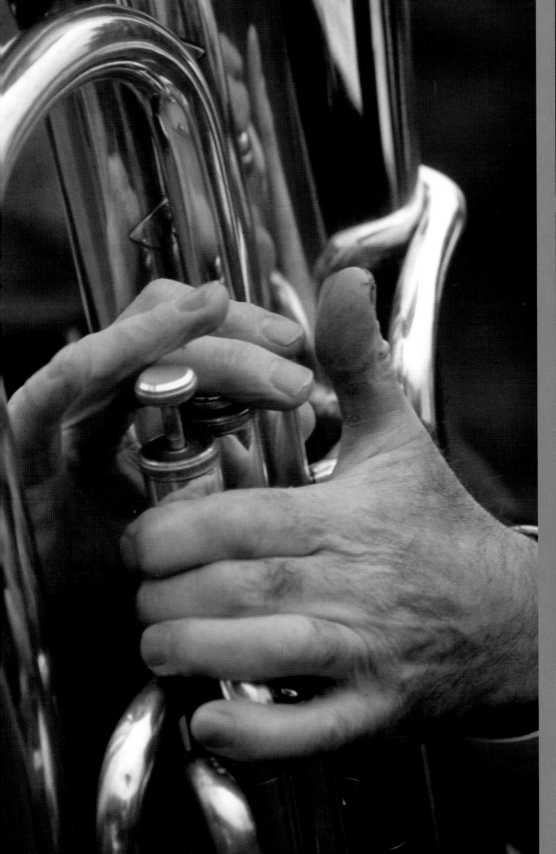
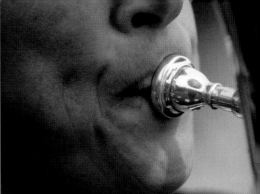
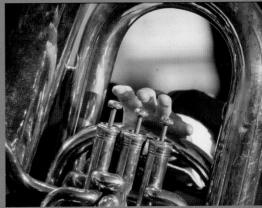
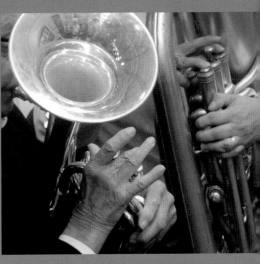

At engagements I'd take my camera and hang it on the seat in front of me. If I had a sixteen-bar rest, I'd put down my instrument and pick up the camera to grab some close-ups from within the band. I was particularly interested in pictures of rustic fingers flying over the valves.

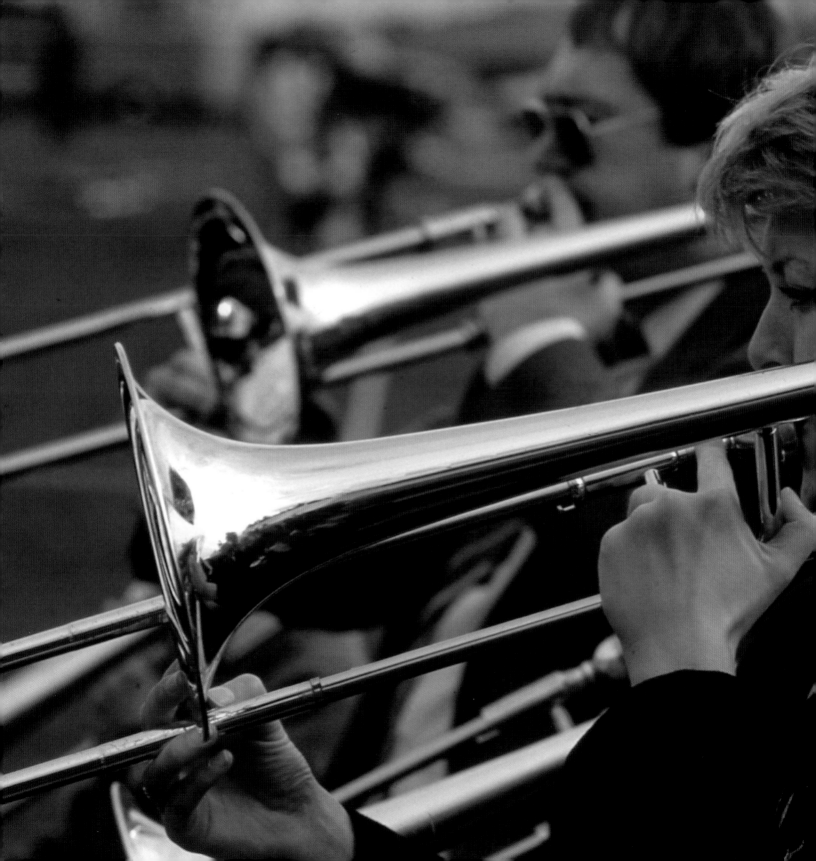

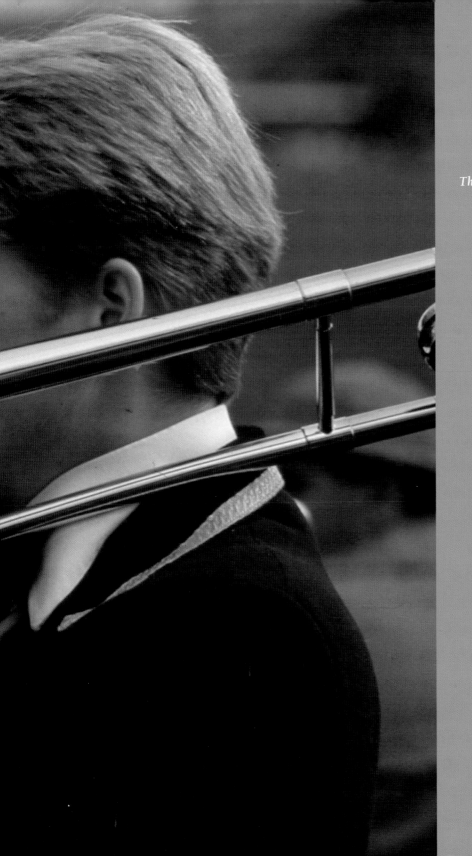

The trombone section.

full moon, a sparkling dusting of snow on the hills, and a starry sky is pure magic.

An editorial in the *Teesdale Mercury* in January 1931 penned by "Mercurius" reads:

" *The Dales, and particularly Teesdale, have always been noted for their musical capabilities and for their brass bands.*

What better music could wake the stillness of the night at the festive season than that of our local instrumentalists playing the songs and choruses and hymns of olden times, stirring memories of earlier days. Long may our local bands continue to give us the best results of their efforts, and long may the spirit of harmony prevail among the hearers. **"**

And so the tradition continues to thrive today, much loved by the dales folk, and celebrating all that is good about village banding: the fun, the camaraderie, and the joy of making music, Thomas Hardy style.

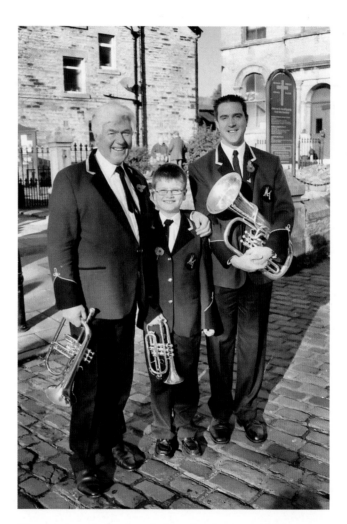

Three generations: Grandad on flugel, my son Dan on euphonium, and his son Alex, aged nine, on his first outing at Remembrance Day in Middleton.

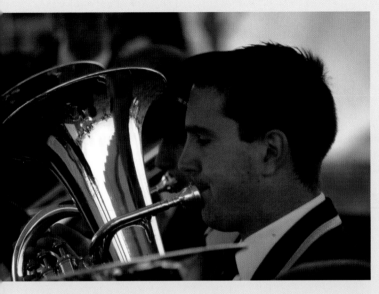

Dan on euphonium.

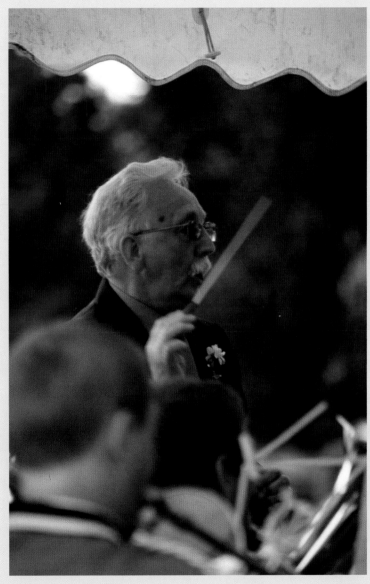

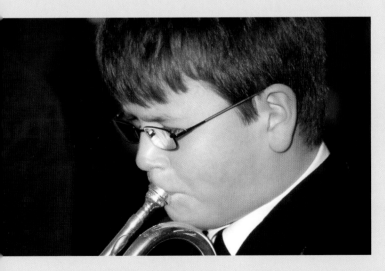

Alex on cornet.

The maestro.

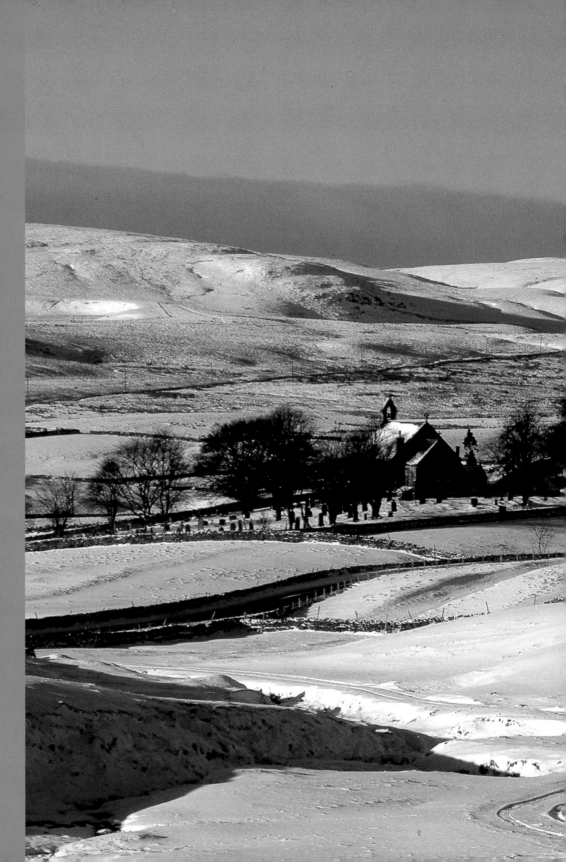

The church of St James the Less where the band play for the service of nine lessons and carols on Christmas Eve. Emerging from the church at nine o'clock to see a full moon, a sparkling dusting of snow on the hills, and a starry sky is pure Christmas magic.

4 Get Ready for the Judgement Day

Yet another heavy shower had passed without dampening the spirits of the good folk attending the village carnival.

Half a dozen Labradors, a beagle, a Bedlington terrier and a host of dogs of uncertain parentage paraded around the show ring. I stood in the middle with the unenviable task of choosing the Dog with the Waggiest Tail!

There were several main contenders for the title. Whilst some did not wag at all, others wagged, waved, and gyrated their tails with gusto. I needed to devise a tie-break. I marshalled the competitors into a straight line facing me, told them to turn through 180 degrees so that all the tails faced me, and exhorted the owners to encourage a prize-

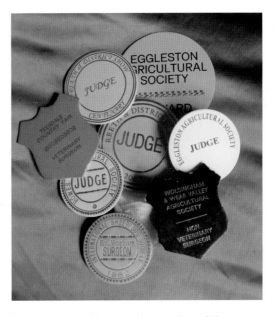

My collection of badges from a few of the events where I've been "Hon Vet" or done some judging.

winning wag. The result was fantastic. At last I had a clear winner. The wag of Yo-Yo the yellow Labrador was outstanding. The tail was a flurry of activity, whilst the hind legs, hips, loins, and chest seemed to be involved too. Not only the tail was wagging: the whole dog was wagging too.

The next classes were just as difficult. I had to choose the dog with the most appealing eyes, dog in best condition, best cross-bred, best pedigree, most unusual pet, and an overall champion. At the end I was happy that I had taken my task seriously, made the right decisions, and had a lot of fun. More importantly, the entrants and spectators had enjoyed it too.

I love being involved in the village carnivals and agricultural shows. They are such an integral part of country life; a statement of belonging to a rural community. My involvement may be simply the "Hon Vet" duties, or I may also be asked to be a judge in an animal or photography section. Many years ago, as the village band strode out at the head of the carnival procession, I resolved to join their ranks at some point. Eventually the opportunity presented itself, and my modest mastery of the flugel horn has graced many a carnival procession since then. Thus at some events I have

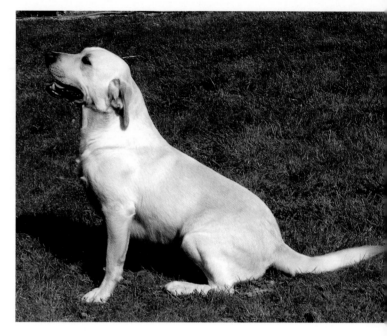

Yo-Yo, the dog with the waggiest tail.

a dual, or even triple role—Hon Vet, judge, and bandsman.

The multiple roles can have quite amusing consequences.

One year I was asked to perform the opening ceremony and judge the fancy dress competition at our village carnival. It was a tradition that the fancy dress competitors assembled in the playing field for the judging, and were then paraded through the village, led by the band, to the village hall for the opening ceremony. How could I solve the problem of being suitably dressed for both my formal duties and the band procession?

My wife, Chris, came up with the answer. She would stand by with a spare jacket and tie. As soon as I had completed the fancy dress judging, I changed into band jacket and tie to join the band in the procession. Having marched with the band to the village hall I swiftly changed back into "civvies", to perform the opening ceremony. Then it was back into band livery yet again for the afternoon concert. It had been a frantic affair, but no problem for a carnival junkie like me!

It is always fun recollecting the Turner family's contributions to our local event. Arthur and Dan had been decked out over the years as Batman and Robin, cowboys, Arabs, a Tate and Lyle sugar cube, and a tableau from *It Ain't Half Hot Mum*. The inspiration was always a last-minute affair.

A dual role at a large local event had amusing consequences too.

I had informed the organisers that for most of the day I would be playing in the band, as well as being the Hon Vet. They didn't have a problem with this,

and provided me with a radio telephone, should my professional services be needed. Halfway through the afternoon I was summoned from the bandstand to attend a dog with a damaged leg. The owners were a dear old couple who were very grateful for my prompt, efficient attention, but ever so amused at the Hon Vet turning up in a green jacket with black facings and liberal applications of gold braid. The outfit was completed by white shirt and black tie.

The story found its way into the *Northern Echo* the following week in a superbly written tongue-in-cheek piece, the gist of which was that it must have been a very high-class event where the vet turns out in full livery.

One year I had the honour of being the president of the local agricultural society show. It was indeed a great honour, but the duties on show day were not too onerous. I had to give a speech at the formal lunch on the show field, and present the major trophies. The only other task traditionally delegated to the president was to judge the mounted fancy dress.

This competition happens at the end of show day and it is a high-profile affair attracting many

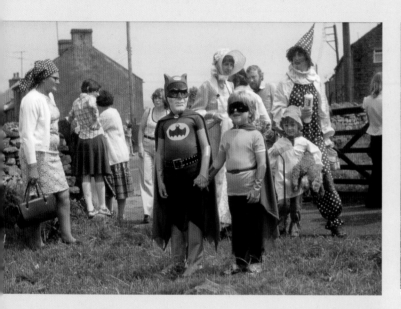

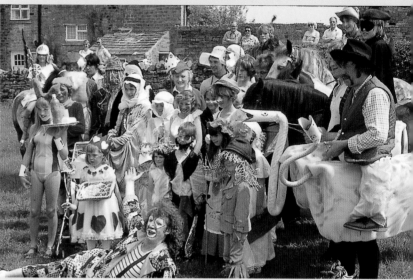

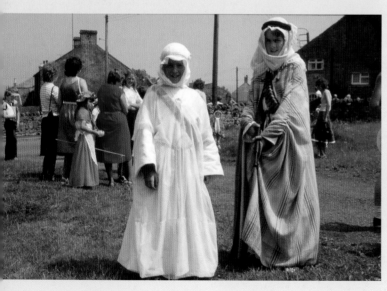

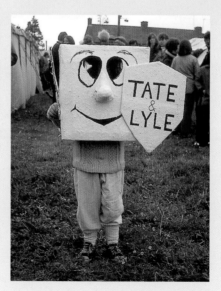

Turner family contributions to the village carnival.

spectators. The outfits are wonderful, and there are usually lots of entries. The children aboard the ponies have a marvellous time, but the parents have a reputation for being fiercely competitive. My steward was a local farmer whom I knew well, and he had been on the show committee for decades.

I asked for any tips he had regarding the judging of this prestigious event, and I shall never forget his reply, delivered with a wry smile.

"Keep your car handy with its engine running!"

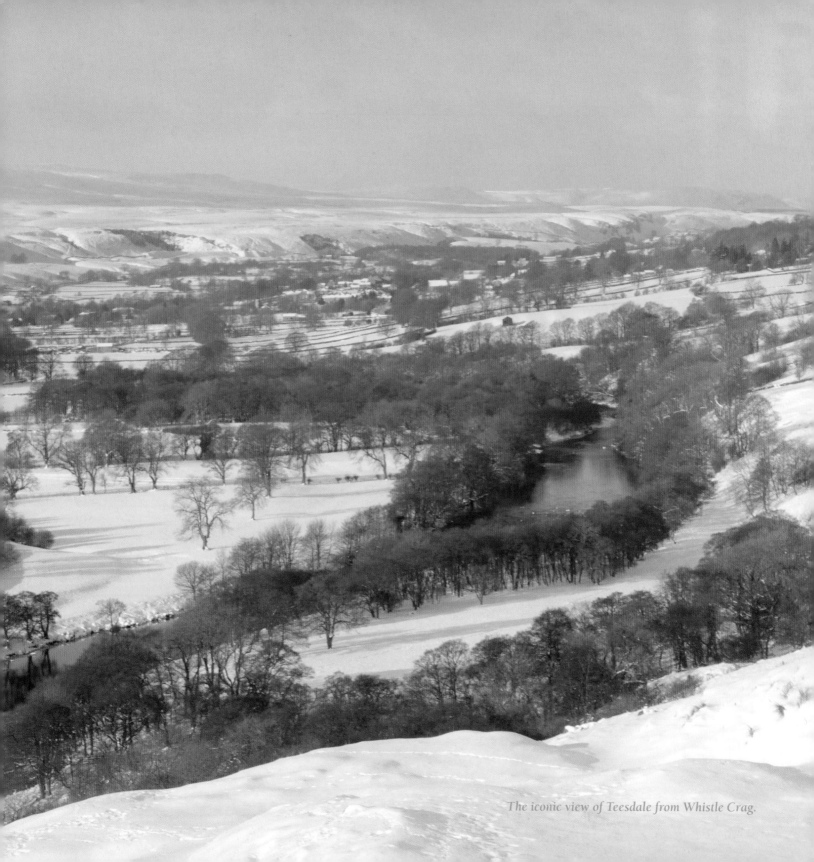

The iconic view of Teesdale from Whistle Crag.

5 The North Wind Doth Blow

(and we shall have snow!)

Travelling 35,000 miles each year in beautiful Teesdale countryside sounds like an idyllic perk in any job.

And so it was.

Over three and a half decades, that adds up to about a million miles, equivalent to driving to the moon and back twice. I know every nook and cranny, or every crook and nanny, if you prefer! I love the landscape, the architecture, the history, the people, and the wildlife.

The big drawback is that six out of every twelve months can be classed as winter. Gordon Manley, a great climatologist who made a study of the Pennine hills between 1932 and 1978, noted that "mean May temperatures were like January temperatures in London, and the dales climate was akin to that at sea level in Iceland."

The stark majestic beauty of the dale clad in fresh snow is awesome, but poses serious problems when one needs to travel from A to B. Over the years I've gained a healthy respect for snow. In such conditions brakes, accelerator, gears, and steering wheel are all used with the lightest of touches.

I'm no hotshot driver, but I do have one party piece that is particularly useful in snow. (It's worth noting that this only works on ice or hard-packed snow. If you try it on tarmac you could wreck your car!) By engaging reverse gear, putting the wheels on full lock, revving hard, and letting out the clutch sharply, the car will pirouette in its own length, facing the way it came. This manoeuvre has saved me from many a sticky situation. It was very useful when a violent and unexpected mid-December blizzard hit the dale.

By late morning the conditions had deteriorated to a white-out. I was at the branch surgery and needed to make the eleven-mile journey to Barnard Castle. I negotiated the notorious Keverstone Bank, and as I passed through the village of Staindrop I felt that I had passed the worst hazards. However, a mile west of the village a snowplough had foundered and I found myself at the tail end of a line of a dozen cars which were stuck behind it.

In white-out conditions this was not a good place to be. I hit every switch on the dashboard. Hazard lights and rear fog-lamps would surely alert the next driver to join the queue, but they didn't. Headlights appeared in my rear-view mirror and the car lurched as the driver saw me. There was no way this fellow would stop. I braced myself for the impact, but the car slewed past me at a

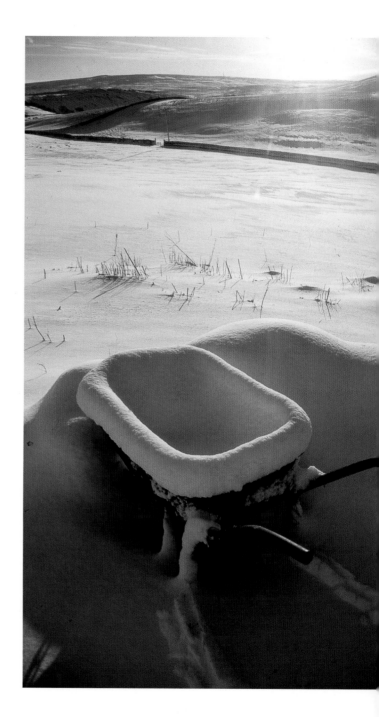

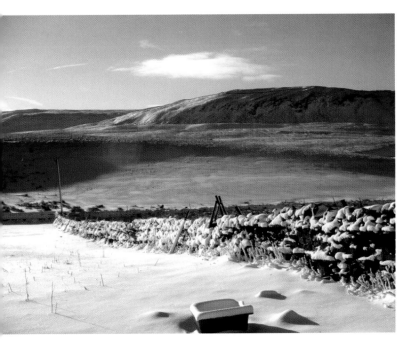

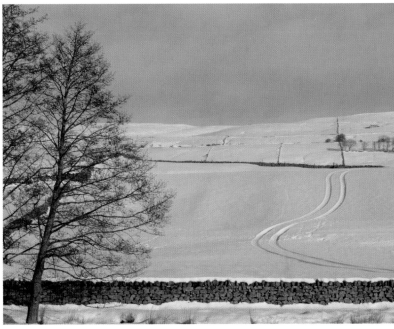

The stark beauty of the dale under a fresh cover of snow.

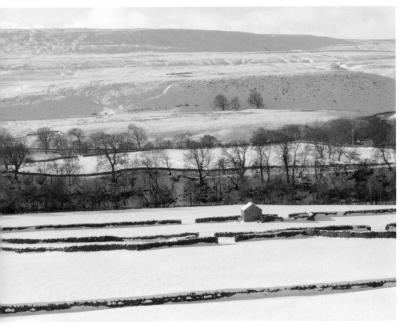

crazy angle. It just missed my off-side wing and embedded itself in a snowdrift at the side of the road.

"I'm not staying here," I thought, and executed my party piece to attain the relative safety of Staindrop.

Once there, I telephoned my colleagues and my family from a call box, giving them the good news (that I was safe and well) and the bad news (that Staindrop was seriously cut off from the rest of the world).

Wondering what to do next, I remembered my invitation from Roy Beadle. Roy was a lovely man who had farmed for many years in the upper dale, just above the great waterfall of High Force. He had retired to a small cottage in picturesque Staindrop a couple of years previously. On my last visit to his farm before he retired, he had said, "If you're ever in Staindrop and have a few minutes to spare, do pop in for a cup of coffee."

So I did.

He was delighted to see me, and although the electricity supply to the village was down, he had a roaring fire, a saucepan of boiling water, and some (as he described it) REAL coffee. We spent a wonderful, convivial afternoon sitting by the fire exchanging stories.

The 30th December 1978 saw the first of four violent snowstorms which crippled communications in the dale for three months. On the night the storm struck we received a call from a remote farm in the upper dale: "We've got a cow that we think is having trouble calving. There's no way you'll get here tonight, but will you try in the morning?"

The following morning we arranged for a four-wheel-drive vehicle to ferry me to a spot as near as possible to the farm. A friend had kindly volunteered to accompany me. This was no journey to be undertaken solo. We packed a rucksack with emergency rations, and everything we might need for a bovine obstetrical case.

The two-mile trek through waist-deep snow was arduous. The calving case, although successful, was physically exhausting (I'll spare you the details). The return trip wasn't much fun either, despite our being fortified with mugs of coffee and slabs of excellent Christmas cake. We had set out at first light and returned after dark. The warm glow of thawing out was accentuated by thoughts of a job well done.

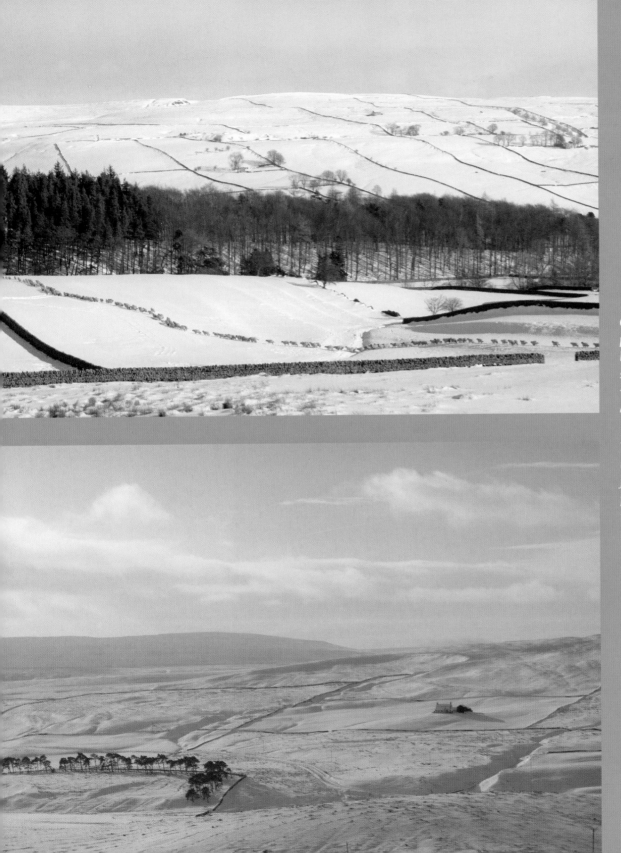

On the extreme left of the picture you'll see a tractor bringing breakfast. The sheep seem to be doing the very British thing of forming an orderly queue.

The upper dale farmers used to stock up with barrels of flour and oatmeal, sacks of potatoes, and sides of bacon in October. People living in such remote spots could be cut off for weeks in the winter.

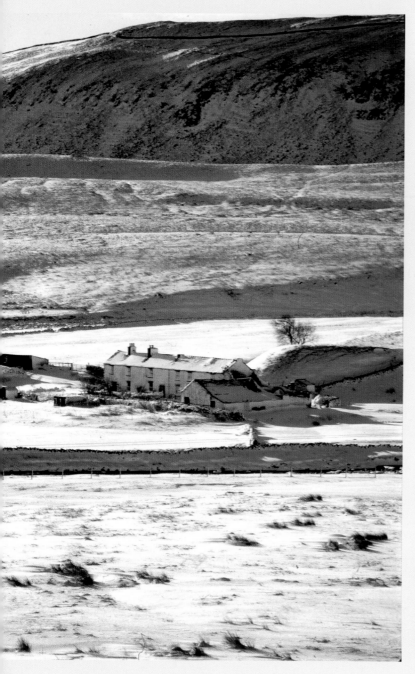

Whey Syke, another isolated dales farm.

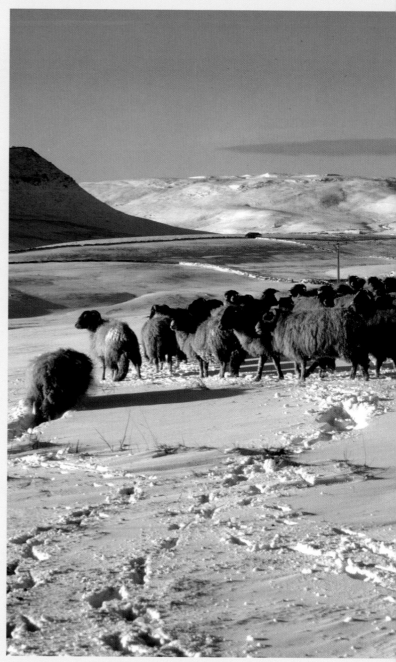

The hardy Swaledale sheep could survive out of doors over winter thanks to a thick weatherproof fleece.

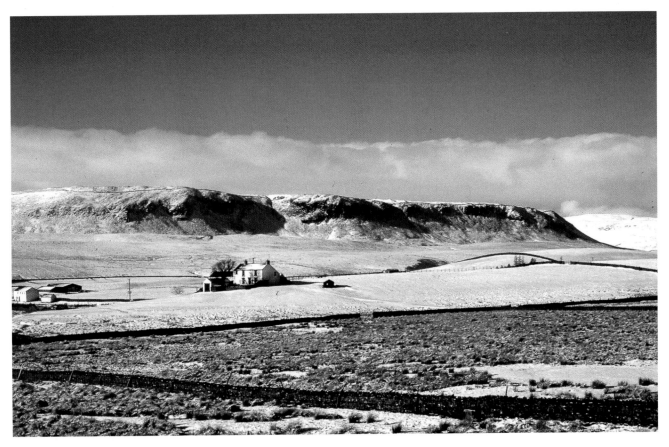

Cronkley Scar, an eighty-metre-high slab of basalt, is thrown into sharp relief by the snow.

Occasionally, on visits to remote farms when the lanes were filled with snow, it would be prudent to leave the car by the side of the road, and travel on foot down the track to the farmhouse. I remember well doing this in Lunedale a few years ago. Having battled my way through deep snow for half a mile and attended my patient, I surveyed the landscape to plan the best route back to the car.

The lanes and fields were filled to wall-top level, but I had a brilliant idea. What if I were to walk along the top of the stone walls that protruded from the snowy blanket, in a sort of tightrope act?

All went well for the first part of the journey. This really was a brilliant idea.

Perhaps it was over-confidence or it could have been a particularly icy patch on the stone wall that led to my downfall. As my foot slipped, time seemed to slow down, like an action replay on *Match of the Day*. Arms and legs spread, I punched a neat hole in the snow and sank about four feet below the surface.

Unable to move, I lay flat on my back gazing at a patch of blue sky shaped exactly like me. It was as though the snow was a thick sheet of gingerbread, and someone had pressed out a life-size gingerbread man.

I lay there and giggled. It was like a scene from a Walt Disney cartoon. It took a great deal of wriggling and squirming before I had room to move in my pit and make vertical headway. With each wriggle, snow fell from above and threatened to bury me. It took ages to extract myself from this predicament.

The farmer had been very thoughtful and watched my precarious progress to ensure my safe return to the car. When I had disappeared and not immediately reappeared, he suspected the worst and forged his way through the snow to my rescue. He arrived just as my head appeared from the hole. I must have looked like the abominable snowman!

6 How My Slide Show Got Afloat

When I arrived in Teesdale in the early 1970s, the wonderful, magical tales of James Herriot were enjoying huge popularity. As a result, it was assumed that all vets were gifted raconteurs with a wealth of stories to tell. Invitations to speak at Women's Institutes and Rotary Clubs came thick and fast, and I found that I enjoyed these engagements.

Being an enthusiastic amateur photographer, I used pictures taken on my rounds to illustrate my talks, so my picture-taking took on a new sense of purpose. It resulted in a huge photo-library covering not only my professional life, but my love of the Pennine Dales. It included the landscape, natural history, the culture, and the life and work of those who live there.

Then suddenly my shows moved from a parochial stage to a global platform, and the new audiences continue to be enchanted by my pictures and stories of dales life.

Here's how it came about.

Many years ago there was a knock on the door of my family home. My mother went to the door to find two strangers there.

"Hi, I'm your cousin Milton from Detroit, and this is my wife, Doris."

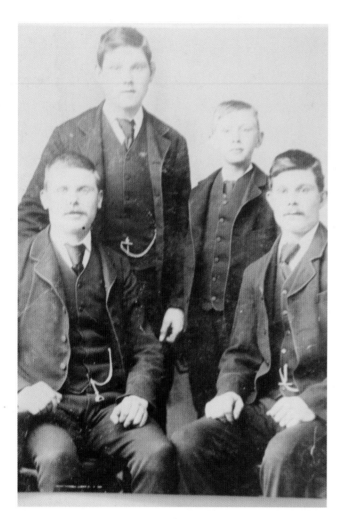

My grandmother's brothers emigrated to the USA in 1910.

You can imagine my mother's amazement. This was the first face-to-face contact between these particular branches of the family in seventy years.

It was in 1910 that four of my mother's uncles emigrated to America. They had been employed at the famous Randolph Colliery, in the Durham coalfield. Life as a coalminer was never easy, and in those days it was positively gruelling, as well as presenting danger to life and limb. It was not surprising that the four had decided to make a fresh start on the other side of the Atlantic.

Some found success farming in Kansas, but Milton's grandfather headed for Detroit, Michigan. It was a good place to seek one's fortune then, as Detroit was nurturing the embryonic motor car industry. That embryo was to evolve into "Motown", home of the giant corporations of Ford, Chrysler, and General Motors. Successive generations worked for these corporations. Milton himself was an engineer with General Motors, and Doris's father was an executive with Chrysler.

There must have been something in the family genes that produced good letter writers. The families kept in constant touch. Throughout my childhood I remember regular letters from America

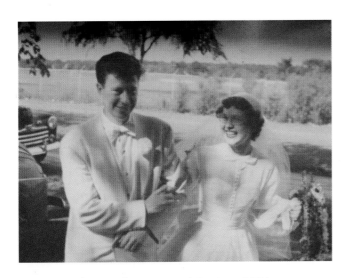

Their grandson, Milton, married Doris in 1956.

In 1996 Milton and Doris came to visit us again, but this time they were celebrating their ruby wedding. To mark the occasion they came over in style on the QE2. They stayed for a week, and after breakfast on the morning they were to leave, Milton made an announcement. It transpired that he had brought with him a selection of back issues of my published works, and presented them to the cruise director, suggesting that his cousin (me) would make a brilliant cruise lecturer.

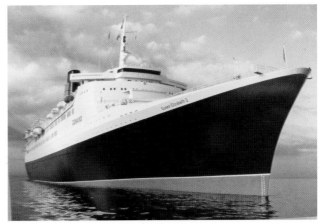

Doris and Milton came to stay with us in 1996. As it was their ruby wedding, they celebrated by crossing the Atlantic on the QE2. Unbeknown to me, they spoke to the cruise director about their cousin who did illustrated lectures.

with enclosed photographs giving fascinating glimpses of life over there, and stamps to be carefully steamed off the envelopes for my stamp album.

Doris and Milton's visit rekindled family connections, and resulted in many get-togethers on both sides of the Atlantic. Doris and Milton were so proud of their roots over here, and I made a subscription for them to a local countryside magazine to which I contributed regularly. They loved the magazine, and in particular waxed lyrical about my contributions.

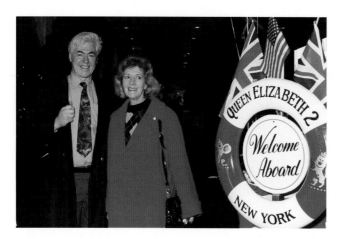

This resulted in a speaking engagement on the QE2 later that year. Chris and I flew to New York and sailed back to Southampton.

The cruise director must have read the magazines because he contacted Milton and urged him to pass on to me the address of Cunard's speakers booking agent.

I obviously had known nothing of this, and could scarcely believe what Milton had done. Our cousins were aware that I had been presenting illustrated lectures to audiences of twenty or thirty for many years, and that I loved doing it. But the thought of addressing hundreds of passengers on one of the great ocean liners was mind-blowing. I could not believe that I would be engaged on the strength of

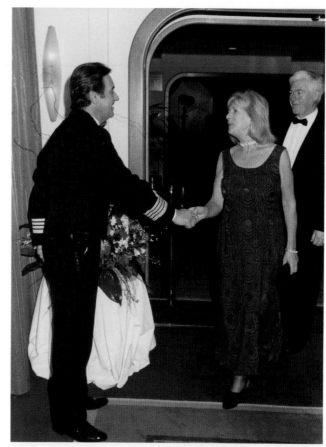

QUEEN ELIZABETH 2   **Photographed on board 2000**

The captain's reception.

some magazine articles and Milton's enthusiasm, so I deferred making the call.

Eventually I plucked up the courage, more out of respect for Milton's efforts than belief in my abilities. And to my surprise, the agency was expecting my call. The cruise director must have spoken to them. I had a most convivial conversation, at the end of which I was given a list of transatlantic crossings, and told to choose any one I wanted.

One is at a distinct advantage when talking about animals and the countryside. Everyone has some interest in those topics. You have only to look at the TV guide to see the popularity of programmes like *Countryfile*, *Supervet*, *Escape to the Country*, *Animal Hospital*, *Wildlife Rescue*, and many others to appreciate the appeal. I must have done well, because Cunard asked me back, and that was the start of a long career as a cruise lecturer.

Since then Chris and I reckon we have visited over a hundred ports in over thirty countries on some wonderful cruise ships. We've seen places we never imagined we'd ever see, such as Mumbai, Rio, Tahiti, Acapulco, and Buenos Aires.

One of the highlights was striking up a friendship with Terry Waite, a lovely man who captured

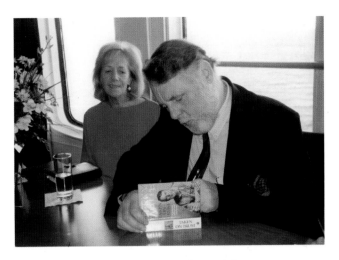

We have struck up acquaintanceships with many interesting fellow lecturers. Here Chris is helping Terry Waite at a book-signing.

the world's sympathy when he was held hostage in Beirut. On another occasion we had a dinner cooked personally by Marco Pierre White.

One of Doris's favourite words is "serendipity", the happy collision of circumstances leading to a delightful conclusion. Serendipity surely played its part in this tale of four coalminers setting off across the Atlantic more than a hundred years ago, resulting in a wonderful friendship which, in turn, was to send Chris and me around the world.

7 How I Was Brought to Book

My interest in the wildlife of the Pennines and my daily journeys over the heather moors led to an interest in the red grouse. Over the space of several years, I amassed a comprehensive photographic record, some of which was used extensively by Saatchi and Saatchi in their advertising campaigns for a well-known brand of whisky. (I'll leave you to work out which one!)

It was such a thrill to see my pictures on bus stops all over the country, and for a while they were everywhere on the London Underground. We even came across images in airports at Schiphol and Prague.

Word of my grouse collection must have spread, for I received a telephone call from Bill Mitchell.

Bill had been editor of *Dalesman* magazine for many years and is one of the most knowledgeable and prolific writers on all matters concerning the rich and unique culture of the dales. The call was because of a brochure that he was producing for a local estate. He needed pictures of the red grouse, and had heard on the grapevine that my library was the definitive source.

I was impressed by his manner, and happily submitted a dozen pictures with my good wishes for the project. I added that there would be no fee, but I would appreciate a couple of copies of the brochure for my scrapbook.

From that initial contact Bill and I became good friends. There were letters and phone calls, and a

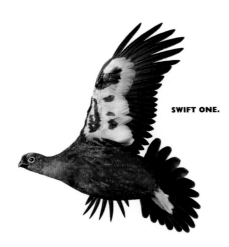

SWIFT ONE.

regular exchange of our latest published work. Our mutual enthusiasm for the culture and wildlife of this part of the world forged a strong link, although it would be many years before we would meet, face to face.

Years later I received a letter from the management of Dalesman Publishing, enquiring about the content of my photo-library, and asking to see some examples of my published work. My friend Bill had been consulted about the feasibility of producing an illustrated book on the subject of life on a dales hill farm and, being familiar with my work, had suggested that I might be a fertile source of material.

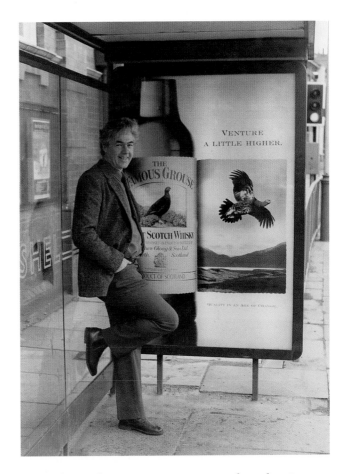

Some of my red grouse pictures were used to advertise a "famous" brand of whisky. This resulted in my being contacted by Bill Mitchell, renowned dales author and long-time editor of Dalesman *magazine, who needed some grouse portraits. We became firm friends, and this friendship was responsible for my being commissioned by* Dalesman *to write and illustrate a book on hill farming.*

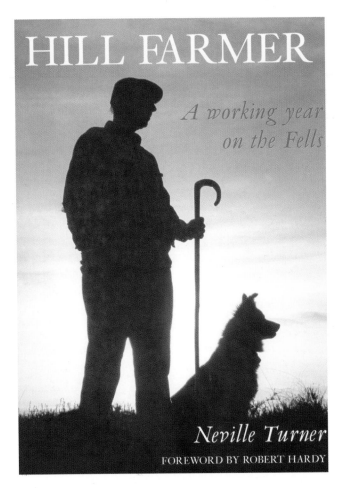

The cover of Hill Farmer. *I did the shoot at sunset on Barningham moor. Bill Bell, a shepherd and friend, made a great model.*

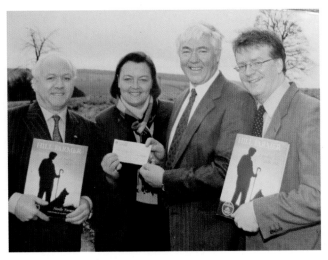

Dalesman decided to make a donation to the Royal Agricultural Benevolent Institution from each copy sold, in the wake of the Foot and Mouth crisis. Robert Flanagan, general manager of Dalesman Publishing, is on the right of the picture.

Some time later, my wife, Chris, and I travelled to Dalesman HQ in Skipton to spend a convivial afternoon at the boardroom table giving a slide presentation. It was a super afternoon and the book was given the go-ahead, but the icing on the cake was that it was my first meeting with my long-time friend, Bill. He did not disappoint: a gentle, knowledgeable character with a certain dignity and a lovely sense of humour. It is a privilege to call him a friend.

If I'd had to orchestrate my first month of retirement I couldn't have done better. To be let loose with my camera and eighty rolls of film (digital photography was in its infancy) was like a chocoholic being let loose at Cadbury's.

Two and a half thousand frames later I'd spent a morning with a mole-catcher, been heather-burning, muck-spreading, foddering sheep, stone-walling, and lime-spreading. I'd documented calvings, caesarean sections, vaccinating stock, dosing sheep, and clipping out cattle for the sale ring. I'd even been on a nature walk with the pupils of a rural school. Anything and everything to do with the dales was fair game for my camera.

As the deadline approached, Dalesman informed me that Bill had been ill and had not been able to complete the words for the book. They asked if I could take over, and by superhuman effort, I rattled off 25,000 words in twenty-one days.

The launch was a splendid affair. Dalesman had hired Ripley Castle for the event, which was shared with the launch of Sir Bernard Ingham's books on Yorkshire churches and castles.

Freddie Trueman was there, and Sir Bernard, in his address, said that it was a pity Denis Healey wasn't

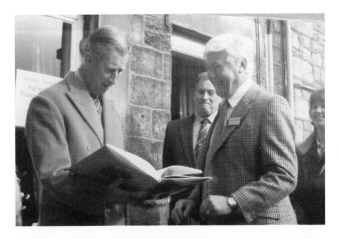

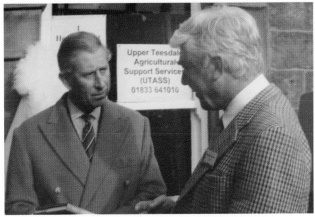

His Royal Highness The Prince of Wales is a great supporter of British farming, and when he visited the Upper Teesdale Agricultural Support Services I was asked to present him with a copy of my book.

there too. If he had been, Freddie, Denis, and Sir Bernard would have displayed the definitive trio of exuberant Yorkshire eyebrows.

Freddie Trueman purchased several of my books, and asked me to inscribe one for himself and his wife. I couldn't resist a broad smile at the thought of the day I met cricketing legend Fred Trueman and HE asked for MY autograph!

The whole project had been a delight, from picture selection and captioning, through proofreading, and eventually holding a copy of my magnum opus in my hands. There followed promotional events and book signings. There are some wonderful memories.

Looking back, we have to thank the late and much missed Alf Wight, author of the James Herriot tales, the Women's Institutes of the North Pennines, and a serendipitous friendship with the remarkable Bill Mitchell for being the catalysts that resulted in my very personal record of the life of the hill farmer.

8 Big Luigi and the Bad Tooth

Without doubt, Luigi was the biggest animal I have ever been called upon to treat—a ton and a half of Chianina bull. He was a magnificent specimen of the breed, all white, but with dark, smouldering eyes, a clue to his fiery Latin temperament.

Colin, his owner, had called me earlier to say that the bull had not eaten properly for several days, and now, looking at him, it was easy to see that the problem was in the mouth. Uneasy tongue and jaw movement coupled with a dribble of saliva from the corner of the mouth were the telltale signs. He was rather ferocious at the best of times, but with the pain of toothache adding to his normal anti-social demeanour, he was positively dangerous.

The Chianina, an Italian breed, was a relatively new introduction to this country. The demand for larger-framed beef cattle had prompted the importation of the Charolais from France in the 1950s. The trickle turned into a veritable spate as Limousin, Simmental, Belgian Blue, and Blonde d'Aquitaine all played their part in displacing the Hereford and Aberdeen Angus.

The Italian contingent comprised Romanola, Piedmontese, and Chianina, so, in the broad face of history, it was not so unusual that I should be standing, on a bright June morning, confronted by three thousand pounds of macho Italian manhood.

Before I could check my diagnosis, Luigi had first to be caught and sedated. Only a fool would have entered his pen to secure his head with a halter. Aggressive snorting and pawing the ground with his forefeet clearly showed that the bull did not appreciate our efforts on his behalf. Colin solved the problem with a long rope. He tied a slip knot to form a lasso, and with the dexterity of a Hollywood cowboy, waved it above his head and loosed it at Luigi. The loop fell neatly around the bull's neck.

Colin and I were joined by his son, Neil, in reeling in our monster catch. With a determination that threatened to herald a hernia, we had the bull within arm's reach, near enough for me to lean over the gate and discharge the contents of a syringe right on target.

The sedative took a few minutes to take effect, but then down he went. I estimated that he would stay that way for about twenty minutes, so I needed to work quickly. Wedging the jaws apart with a metal gag, I soon found the offending tooth right at the back of the mouth. It was loose, but however I manipulated it with my fingers, it stayed stubbornly in the jaw. Frustration was setting in and the minutes were ticking away. Looking back, I loved these adrenalin-filled moments, which necessitated quick thinking, inspiration, and improvisation.

I spotted a huge metal bar leaning against wall and asked Colin to bring it. I also asked Colin if he could find a big brick. The plan was to lay one end of the metal bar against the tooth while Colin struck the other end of the bar with the brick.

There's an old music hall joke with a punch line, "When I nod my head, you hit it," and that was the plan.

Down came the brick. There was a crunch in the mouth. Plan "A" had worked! I handed the tooth to Colin. It would offend no more, and the bull would be able to eat again. All three of us were immensely delighted at the result. I checked the jaw, as Colin had struck a mighty blow, but all was well.

The professional side of the job complete, I decided to photograph the bull before he recovered his senses. Luigi still slept soundly. We manoeuvred his massive head onto a bale of straw and propped it in place. He looked so peaceful.

Young Neil placed his arm around Luigi's gigantic neck as though he was giving him a cuddle, and I lay on the ground, flat on my stomach to get the right angle. Click went the shutter, and as it did so, Luigi's eyes opened. He was awake and looking straight at me. We both sprang to our feet at the same instant. I knew how fast he could move, and I had to be faster. I reached a wall and achieved its seven-foot summit in one gigantic leap. What had never crossed my mind was that I might not be his target.

Colin had come into the yard with three cups of coffee on a tray. Tray and mugs were jettisoned as Neil and Colin fled for their lives down the yard with an angry bull in hot pursuit. I watched the great creature close on the two men. Fortunately the bull had chosen the younger, fitter Neil as his target, and actually overtook Colin halfway down the yard. Neil didn't need to look back to know that the bull was behind and gaining fast, but he reached the gate first and vaulted it as though his legs were spring loaded. Luigi hit the gate with a mighty crash but it held, and all was well.

If we could find some more mugs, we reckoned we deserved that cup of coffee!

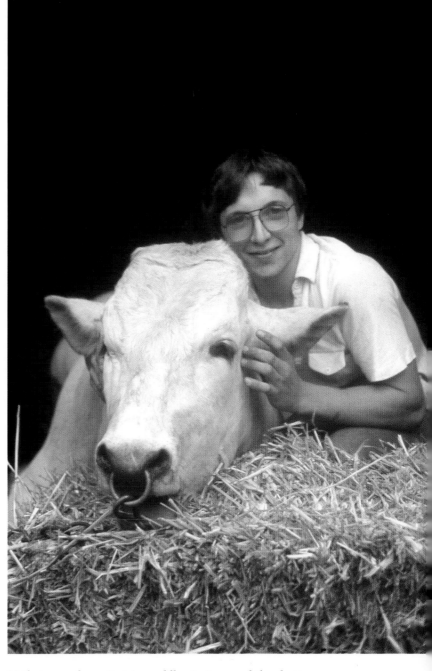

Neil gives a sleepy Luigi a cuddle. As I pressed the shutter, the bull suddenly stood up, and we lost no time in beating a hasty retreat.

9 Pig Tales

Do you remember the case of the Tamworth Two? They were two pigs who escaped while in transit and led their would-be captors a merry dance until at long last they were finally caught. Their escape from their trip to the abattoir was fortuitous, for huge press coverage endeared them to the nation, and they spent the rest of their days as happy and much-loved residents of an animal sanctuary.

We nearly had a repeat performance recently.

A colleague of mine teamed up with a neighbour to purchase two piglets. The aim of the project was to rear the pigs in traditional manner and fill their freezers with wholesome, organic, full-of-flavour pork. The exercise was a great success, but it was not without incident. Their part-time pig-keeping turned out to be, shall we say, eventful.

In particular the loading of the pigs for their final journey led to a couple of fugitives at large in the village. But for a willing bunch of passers-by, the pigs could now be leading a feral existence, grubbing up acorns, beech mast, and roots in the Teesdale woodlands.

There were other incidents.

One night, in the village pub, the landlord happened to mention that he had a barrel of beer that had passed its sell-by date. Our two part-time swineherds, knowing of pigs' fondness for "the juice of the barley", readily took the dated stock and fed it to their charges from time to time as a treat. One day, however, they overdid it. The pigs collapsed in a stupor. At one point they thought the pigs were dead. However, after twenty-four hours' sleep, the pigs awoke and carried on as normal with no sign of a hangover.

The problem is not a new one. Here's a chap who thought he'd killed his pigs too.

Diarist and Norfolk farmer James Woodforde recorded the following on 15 April 1778:

❝ Brewed a vessell of strong beer today. My two large piggs, by drinking some beer grounds got so amazingly drunk by it, that they could not stand and appeared like dead things almost. I never saw piggs so drunk in my life. ❞

During the eighteenth and nineteenth centuries the large breweries and distilleries of London, instead of discharging their waste into the Thames, hit on the idea of using it to feed to pigs. It proved a lucrative exercise. Yearling pigs from all over the country were brought to the capital and fattened for five or six months on the spent grains.

Large-scale pig production declined, but at the same time it became popular for peasants to keep

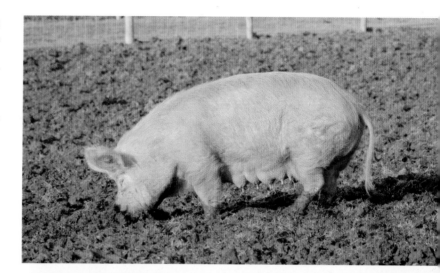

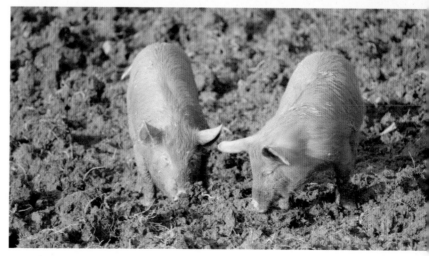

Tamworths are a traditional British breed. Mother and babies are doing what pigs do best: using their snouts to see what they can turn up in the grass roots.

There's a saying, "happy as a pig in muck". There's plenty of muck here, and the pig's benign smile would suggest that it's very happy.

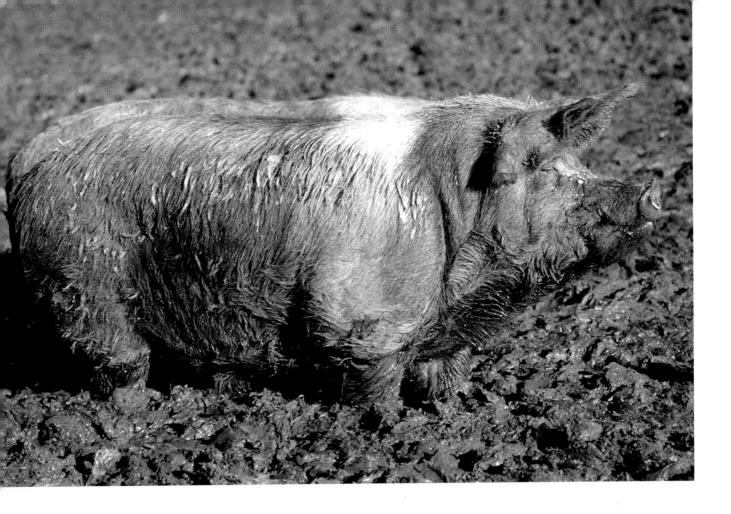

one or two pigs. These were housed for most of the time, and fed mainly on household waste, which suited admirably the species' omnivorous habit. Markham, writing in the seventeenth century, describes "the husbandman's best scavenger, and the housewife's most wholesome sink: for his food and his living is by that which would rot in the yard and make it beastly". Our Teesdale pig-keepers found that very little was consigned to the compost heap while their porcine pals were with them. On one occasion there was a failure on baking day and the pigs were delighted to dispose of a chocolate cake and two dozen meringues.

Small-time pig-keeping endured for hundreds of years. When I first entered practice in the 1960s it was still a common system of husbandry. Many of my patients were to be found on smallholdings or in sheds at the bottom of allotments. Dales farmers, too, often kept one or two pigs for their own use.

Professionally these pigs were a challenge. Although pigs are rarely aggressive, restraining and examining a pig of any size that does not want to be restrained and examined, is virtually impossible. Added to that, the squeals of a protesting pig that is becoming more and more unco-operative builds to an ear-drum-splitting crescendo.

There was, however, one disease that was easy to diagnose: Erysipelas. The patient would be feverish and lying quietly; no high-speed deafening chase around the pig pen here. Large diamond-shaped spots were everywhere on the skin surface. You could even diagnose this disease in a dark cobwebby shed, for the blotches were raised and quite obvious to the touch as one stroked the pig's skin. Although the condition looked grave, the response to a large dose of penicillin was spectacular: a Lazarus-type revival if there ever was one.

There are dozens of pig diseases, but a cynical colleague of mine, fed up with waving his stethoscope at a fast-disappearing pig, announced that there were only two pig diseases: Erysipelas, and *not* Erysipelas.

Maternity cases, too, were different. A sow can produce up to about twenty piglets in a single litter. I've spent many a night waiting for the next baby to move down the uterus into a position where I could effect delivery. Occasionally the sow, having completed delivery of all the little ones, would become aggressive, even killing her own newborn piglets.

Interestingly, one of the old remedies for this was to present her with a few pints of beer, especially if it was fortified with a drop or two of whisky. She couldn't resist the drink, and it usually had the same effect as witnessed by our amateur pig-keepers when they overdid their benevolences to their two charges.

In the last thirty years or so, the veterinary surgeon has met a new and fascinating piggy patient, the Vietnamese pot-bellied pig. A thousand years ago these pigs were kept as pets (and as the occasional meal) in South-east Asia and China. In the 1950s they were introduced to some European zoos as a curiosity, and from there, their popularity took off.

Whilst I, personally, would not be excited by sharing my house with a pig, there are many who have found the VPBP a wonderful pet. They are affectionate, intelligent, and fairly easily house-trained. Everyone who keeps a VPBP seems to be smitten by their good nature.

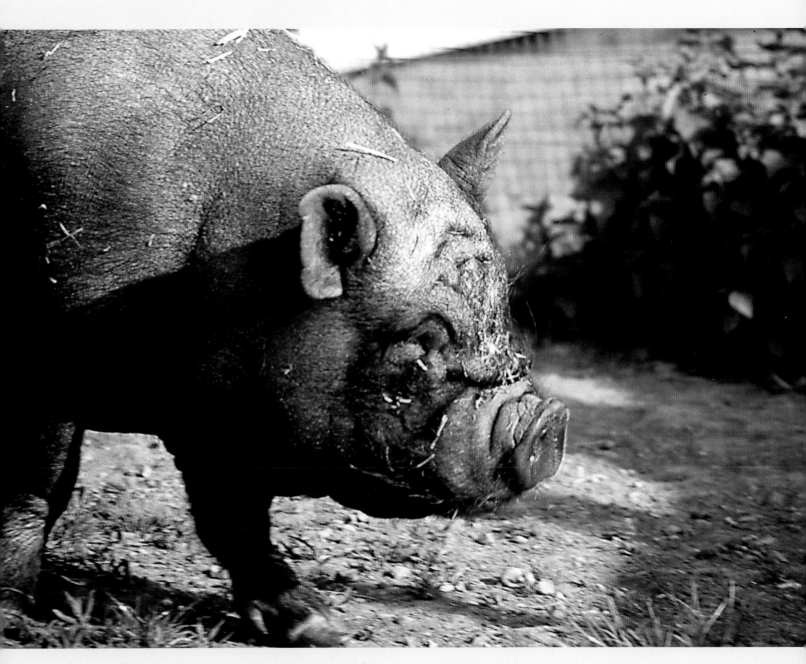

The Vietnamese pot-bellied pig is said to make a wonderful pet.

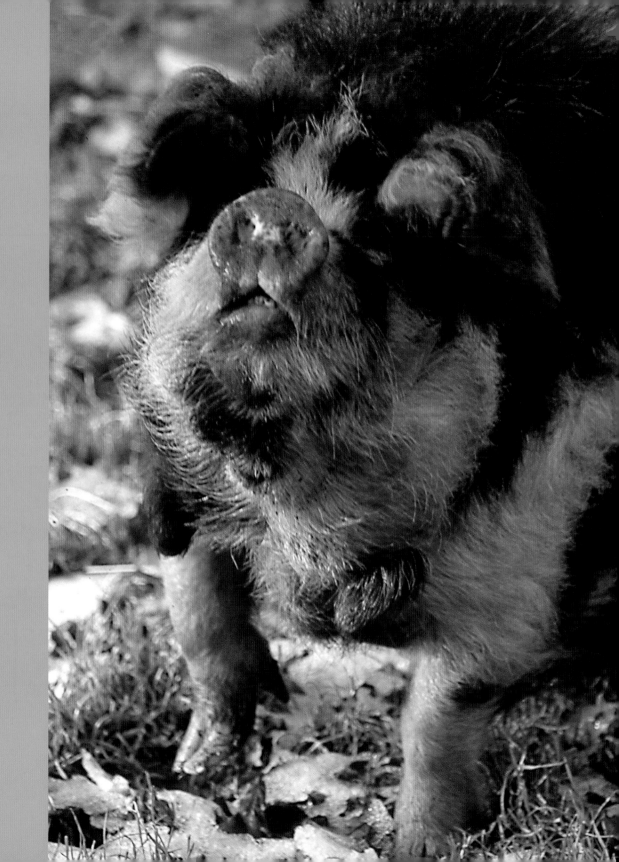

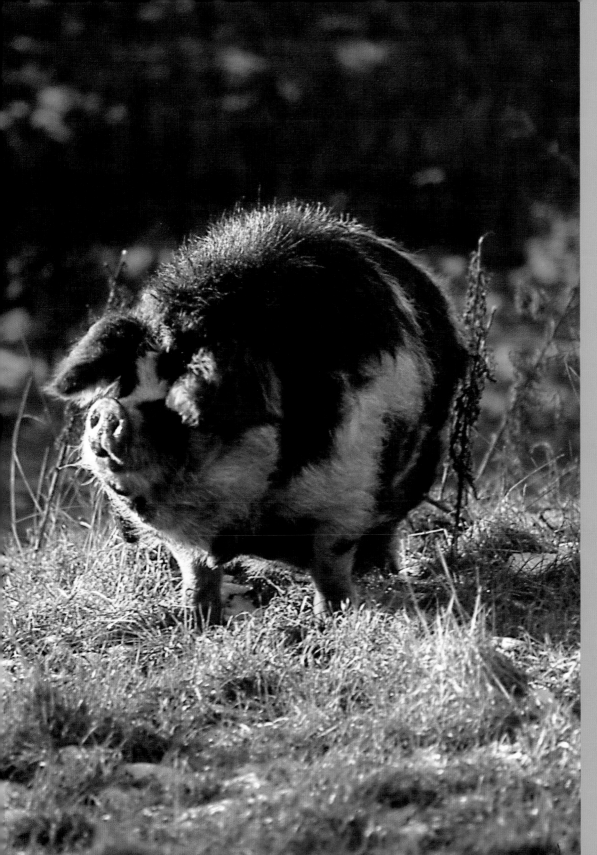

A kunekune pig. A novelty breed with its origins in the Pacific islands.

A receptionist at the practice was one of those smitten. She loved her VPBP dearly, and recounts, without rancour, how when she was out the pig would raid the fridge. This has to be an example of how intelligent a pig can be. The pig would wedge her snout under the seal of the fridge and flick the door back. Once in there she would go through the contents. Her favourite was a jar of Dolmio pasta sauce. She could undo the lid and lick out the contents completely.

When she'd finished with the fridge, she'd attack the larder. Tins were no problem. She'd crunch the tin in her jaws, piercing it with sharp tusks, then suck out the contents.

As I mentioned earlier, pigs are omnivorous, so she didn't even have to read the label!

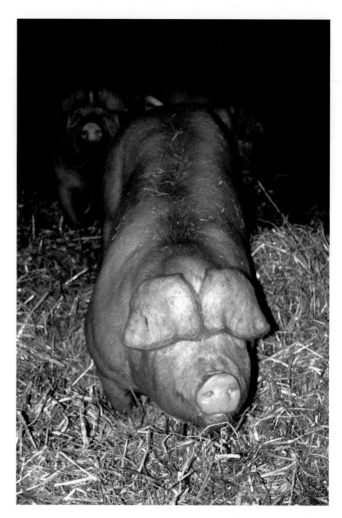

A Pedigree Welsh pig. It looks as though there's a design fault, but the ears aren't always over the eyes.

10 Reflections on the Border Collie

On many occasions in my working day I would arrive at a farmyard that could be likened to the deck of the *Mary Celeste*. A shrill whistle or a double forte "Hallo" was required to raise the farmer's attention from sorting lambs, dipping sheep, or dosing cattle.

On one such occasion I didn't bother to whistle or shout. I knew where the activity would be, so I made my way there through the farm buildings. Emerging from a dark byre into bright daylight, I stood for a moment in the doorway, admiring summer sun lighting the buttercup-laden fields.

And then it hit me!

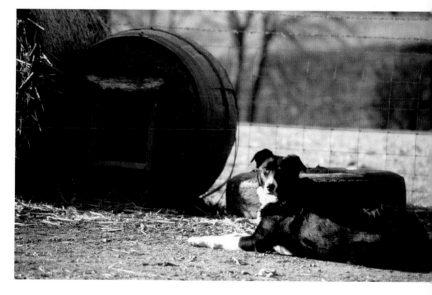

Traditional kennels are rare in the farmyard. Most show ingenious improvisation, such as this elegantly converted wooden barrel.

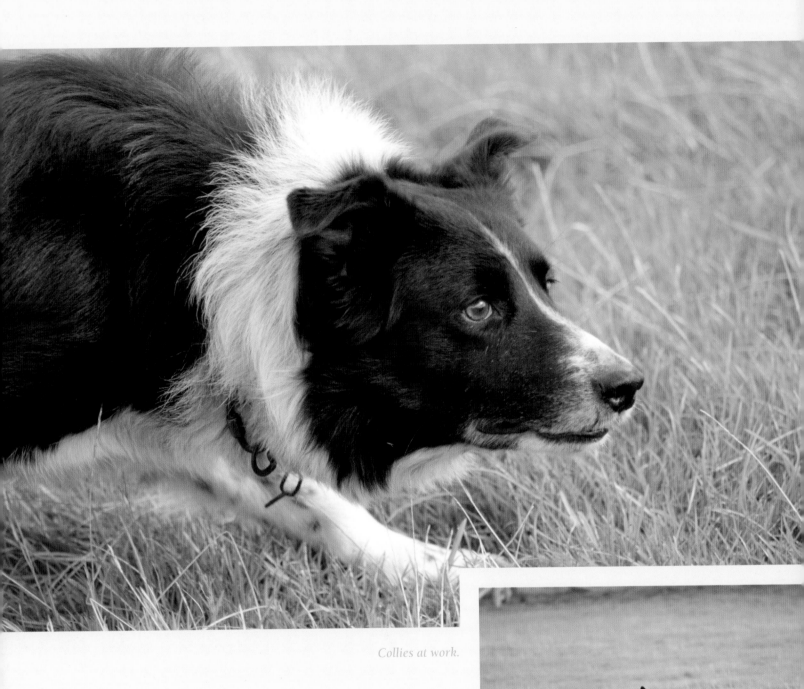

Collies at work.

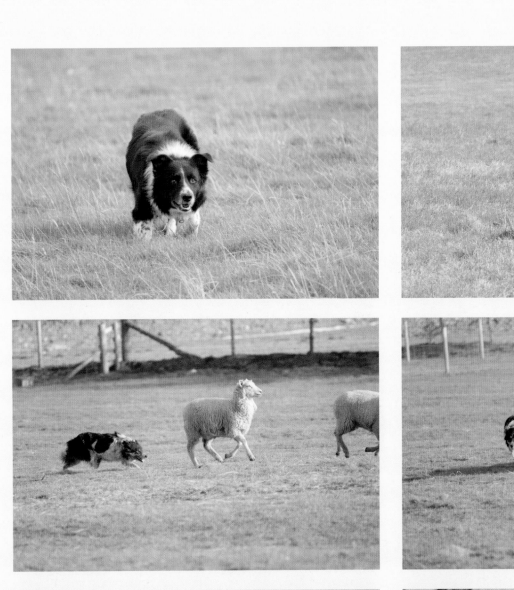

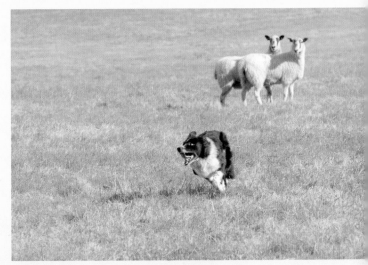

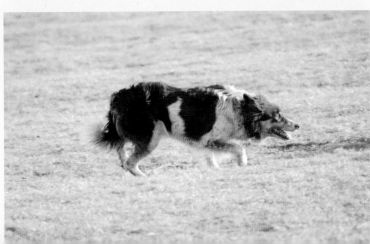

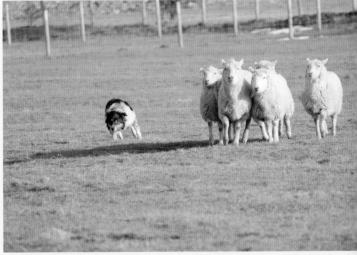

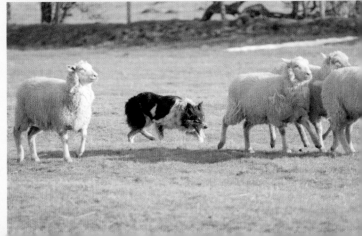

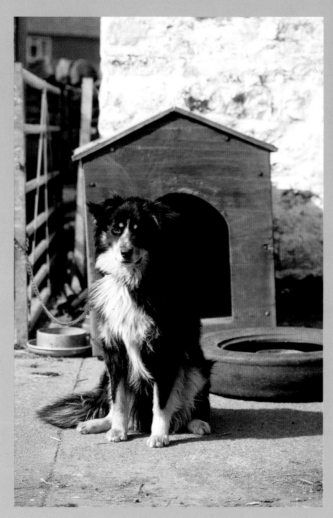

A good-looking dog with a smart, traditional kennel.

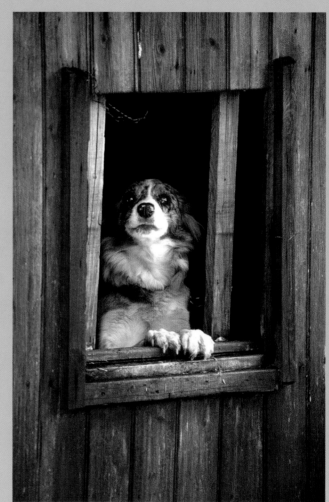

This fellow has a hen house all to himself and seems very happy watching the world go by as he leans on the windowsill.

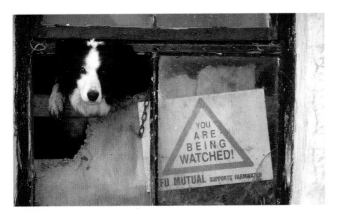

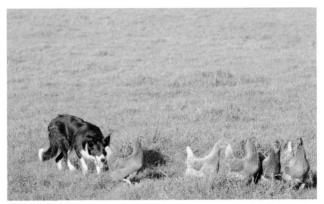

Where there isn't an available kennel, the collie is usually kept in the cowshed. It's good if there's a window so that he can keep an eye on what's going on in the farmyard. The "You are being watched" sign wasn't a set-up. It was purely coincidental.

Blissfully unaware, I had been silently stalked by a collie dog. He chose the perfect moment for the attack. His target was static, beautifully silhouetted, and framed by the byre door. In a split second he struck and retreated into the shadows from whence he had come. I was left in a state of shock, with teeth-marks on one buttock and a large piece missing from the seat of my trousers.

On another occasion, at a different farm, I noticed a collie dog getting very excited about something under my car. I assumed that he was having a bit of sport chasing a farm cat, and had cornered it there. A loud and angry hiss confirmed my suspicions.

Even when I had to stop to change a flat tyre halfway back to the surgery, the truth did not dawn on me. It was only when the repair man found a set

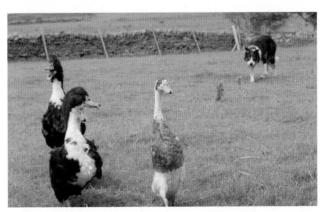

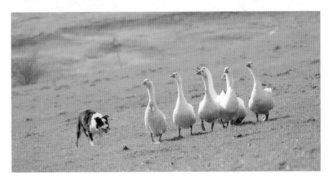

The collie's herding instinct is so strong that they will seize the opportunity to herd anything. Here we see them at work with chickens, ducks, and geese. I've seen them working on turkeys, pigs, and even children!

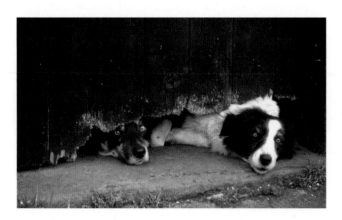

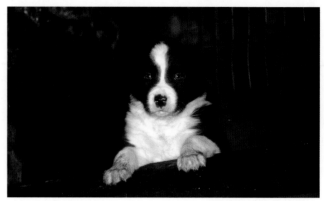

Where there's no window to look through, you can take a strip off the bottom of the door. If you're the sociable type, you can make it big enough for your pal to join you.

Collie pups are very special, full of energy and with a great sense of fun, but with a serious side to their nature, as if they know they'll have a job to do when they grow up.

of teeth-marks in the wall of the tyre that I realised what had happened. The hiss I had heard wasn't that of an angry cat!

Back at the surgery I related the tale to my colleagues. It transpired that two of them had had flat tyres after visits to that farm in recent weeks. A polite phone call was made asking the farmer to lock up his dog when expecting visitors, and the problem was solved.

In spite of the occasional bad experience, most of my contact with the border collie is a joy. I am fascinated by the different sizes, shapes, temperaments, and colours that occur within one breed. It is an indication that this is a dog bred primarily for its working ability.

It was in the hills where the Pennines meet the Cheviots in a massive T-junction, that border shepherds refined the ancient herding dogs into a breed physically and temperamentally perfect for their hill-farming needs. The result of their efforts was the border collie, although that name did not come into general use until 1916.

I must have driven into a dozen farmyards on most working days, and usually the first living thing I saw was the collie dog. Most were friendly. Experience taught me to recognise the ones that weren't.

I am intrigued by the variety of architecture in collie accommodation. Kennels vary from downright primitive to the height of sophistication. And where there is no purpose-built kennel, improvisation is the order of the day. The ingenuity of the dales farmer never ceases to amaze me. As long as the accommodation is waterproof, draught proof, and well bedded, the dog is happy. Oak-staved barrels, oil drums, and disused water tanks may all be called into service.

The collie needs to be fed well for the job he has to do, and the advent of dried all-in-one diets has ensured good nutrition. Before the advent of such foods, a traditional menu was flaked maize and milk. In spite of its popularity, this was a poor diet, deficient in many essential elements. It gave rise to a condition known as "black tongue", characterised by oral ulceration. Fortunately it was readily treatable by an injection of vitamins and some sound advice on feeding.

The modern border collie is a much-loved friend and an indispensable part of the team on a dales farm. No better description has been written than that penned by Robert Burns in his poem, "The Twa Dogs":

> He was a gash an' faithful tyke
> As ever lap a sheugh or dyke.

> His honest sonsie bawsn't face
> Ay gat him friends in ilka place.
> His breast was white, his touzie back
> Weel clad wi' coat o' glossy black,
> His gaucie tail wi' upward curl
> Hung ower his hurdies wi' a swirl.

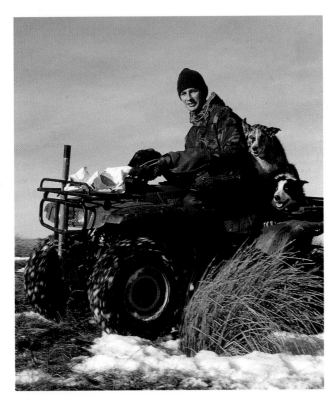

Collies can run all day, but they are bright enough to know that it's easier to hitch a lift.

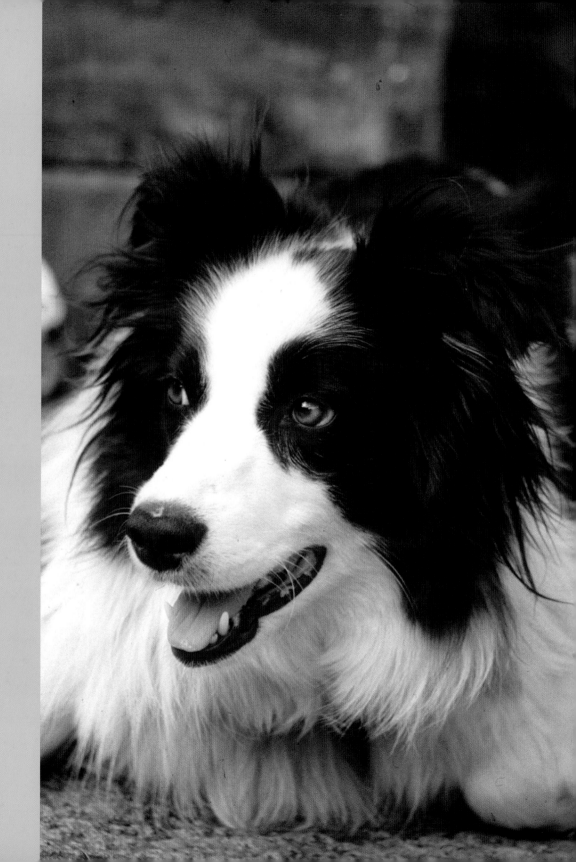

*Portraits of three
good-looking collies.*

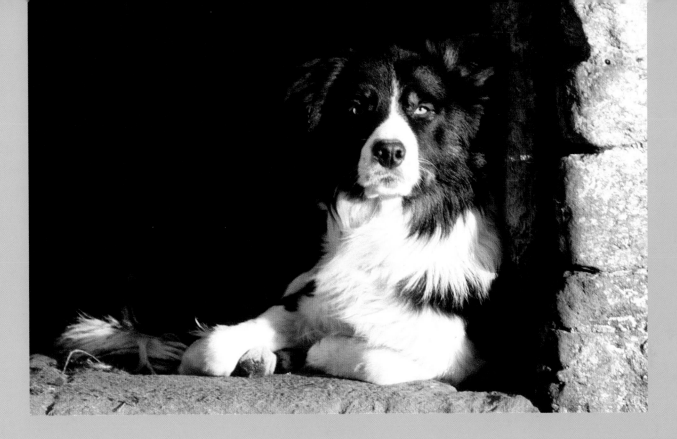

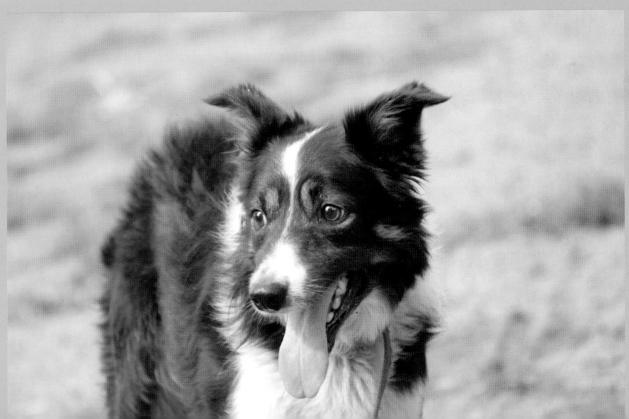

11 All Wired Up for the Operation

"Every day you'll see something new. It may not even be in the textbooks but you'll have to sort it out."

These words, spoken by my mentor when I was "seeing practice" as a student, came back to me as I stood in a byre surveying a cow with six feet of electric fencing wire protruding from her mouth. A herd of bullocks had stampeded through an electric fence earlier in the day, breaking the wire and leaving the loose ends lying on the ground. The cow must have taken up one of the loose ends with a mouthful of grass.

Cows are not blessed with the highest of IQs, and are fairly indiscriminate feeders. Instead of spitting out the offending object, she had continued munching and taking in the wire like a never-ending piece of spaghetti.

The farmer, spotting the predicament, had cut the wire and called the vet.

Logic dictated the initial stages of my investigation. The cow's head was secured with a halter. A metal gag was then wedged between her molar teeth to hold the jaws apart. Sleeves rolled up. My hand followed the wire over the tongue, through the pharynx, and straight down the oesophagus. A gentle tug confirmed my worst suspicions. The other end of the wire was securely fixed somewhere in the cow's stomach, or should I say stomachs, for there are four of them and they're all big! This was a case for surgery.

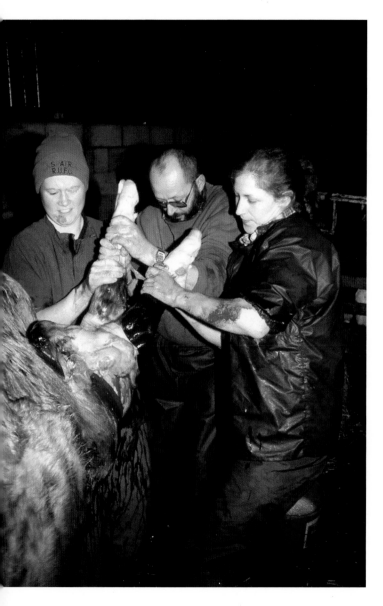

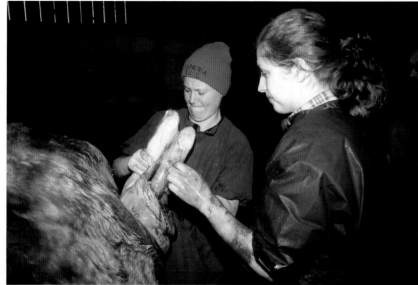

Delivery of a calf by caesarean section is a spectacular sight, especially when one considers that it is performed under local anaesthetic, and the patient is totally unaware of what's going on in her left flank.

Abdominal surgery in the cow is usually performed under local anaesthesia, with the patient in the standing position. The left flank is scrubbed and shaved before a vertical incision is made between the last rib and the upper thigh. Anything less than perfect anaesthesia will result in pain (not only to the cow, but also to the right kneecap of the surgeon as the patient registers her disapproval with a sharp kick from her left hind foot).

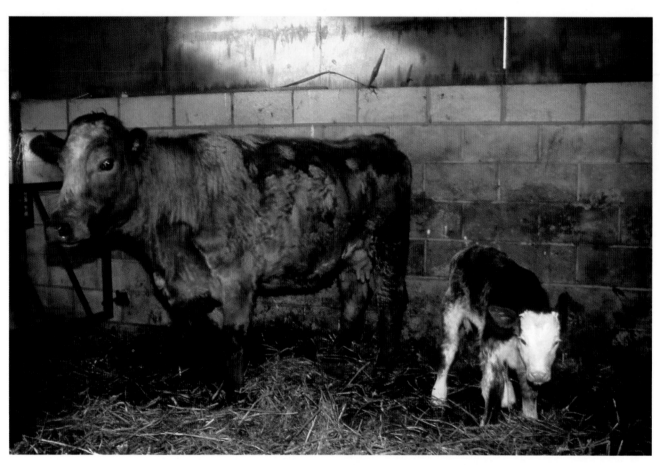

Job satisfaction. Twenty-four hours later, mother and her big calf are doing well. One can scarcely see the surgical wound.

In this case all went well and the abdomen opened with the patient blissfully unaware of my interference. The rumen, the largest of the four stomachs, is easily located. It's huge. The textbooks tell me that its capacity is fifty gallons. I opened it to reveal its contents, best described as three wheelbarrowsful of chopped grass bound up with an entanglement of fencing wire. It was fairly obvious that all the wire could not be removed in one piece, as it was knotted up with stomach contents, so I had to cut away lengths as I extricated them from the tangled mass. I laid each piece, end to end, along the byre floor.

While I stitched up the cow, the owner returned to the field to pace out the gap in the wire as a check that we had removed it all. He returned to announce that his estimate tallied exactly with the length on the floor: fifty-five feet!

The operation I had performed was really a modification of a technique regularly carried out to retrieve foreign bodies from the bovine stomach.

Cows, as I said, are indiscriminate swallowers of foreign bodies, most of them harmless, but short rigid pieces of wire can cause serious trouble. They tend to drop vertically as soon as they enter the stomach and embed themselves in the wall of the stomach closely applied to the diaphragm. Digestive contractions will then, over a period of time, drive the wire through the stomach wall, through the diaphragm, and straight into the heart.

Once the wire hits the heart, there is nothing that veterinary science can do to save the patient. However, in the early stages of the condition, when the stomach is effectively nailed to the diaphragm, diagnosis is easy and retrieval is straightforward.

Another condition of the bovine abdomen requiring surgery is the LDA, or left displacement of the abomasum. The abomasum is the fourth stomach. Nature's grand design has decreed that it lies on the right side of the abdomen, but occasionally it wanders to the left, rotates, and inflates, causing obstruction of the bowel. There are several techniques that can be used to correct the displacement, but our original one was both simple and spectacular.

Two veterinary surgeons were required, one operating on the left, and the other on the right. Both would anaesthetise the flank and open the abdomen.

The surgeon on the left would then grasp the abomasum, pushing it down and across the abdominal floor. The second operator, on the right, would then reach across the abdominal floor, grasp the abomasum proffered by surgeon number one, and draw it up to its natural position. There it would be sutured in place to avoid any recurrence.

Viewed from the rear of the cow, the operation must have presented a bizarre sight, with two vets up to

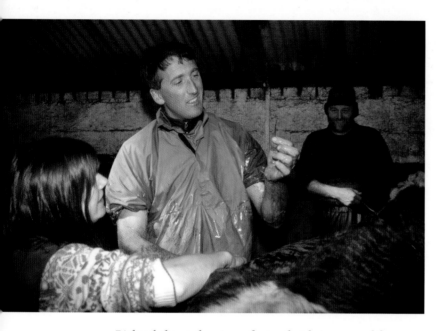

Richard shows the piece of wire that he's removed from a cow's stomach. Left in place it would have proved fatal. The farmer looks highly delighted.

their armpits in a cow's abdomen, and apparently shaking hands in the middle.

The third and perhaps commonest indication for bovine abdominal surgery is the caesarean section. This, again, is accomplished with the cow in the standing position, under local anaesthesia, and via a classic vertical incision in the left flank. The operation takes about an hour: ten minutes to effect delivery, and fifty minutes to put the cow back together.

To call at the farm the next day to find the cow tucking into her hay ration and a big healthy calf sucking vigorously gives a warm glow of job satisfaction.

12 Getting my Goat!

It was 1980 when I first experienced the thrill of seeing one of my pictures published.

Hundreds have appeared in print since then in books, magazines, newspapers, and posters, and it's always a thrill, but seeing the first one remains a special moment. And the subject was a goat called Billy!

I love goats. They are such characters. I always feel that the cat and the goat have an ambivalent opinion of domestication. They have an air of, "Should I choose to do so, I could be totally independent of you, but for the moment I choose to be a part of this relationship."

There is evidence of this, for in many parts of the British Isles there are colonies of goats that have reverted to the feral state, and are quite happy to have done so. Feral goats occur on the Great Orme at Llandudno, in the Cheviot Hills, and in the Western Isles.

1980 marked the centenary of the British Goat Society. A friend who owned a renowned Toggenberg billy goat had been asked by the society for a picture of this goat for inclusion in the centenary yearbook. I, in turn, was asked to take the picture of this famous animal, and was delighted to accept the challenge. Taking pictures of any animal is always a challenge. However, there are limits to how far one can stage manage an animal that refuses to co-operate.

The shoot took place on a knoll on my friend's farm, with low evening sunlight providing perfect conditions. I had calculated that if the goat were

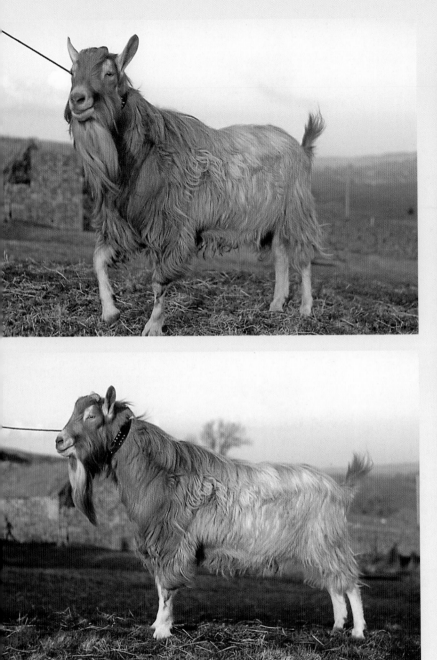

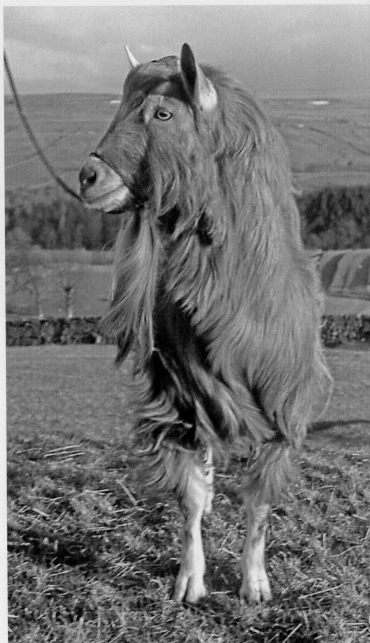

Setting up "Billy" for a portrait was fraught with difficulty . . .

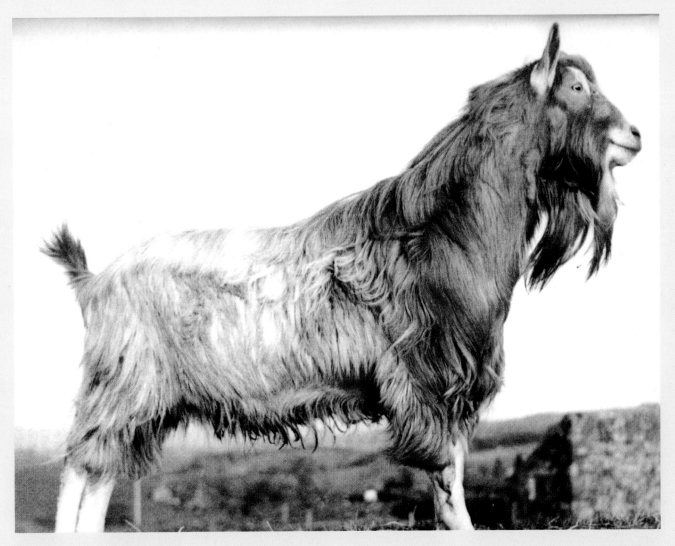

. . . but eventually we succeeded, and here's the picture of him that appeared in the centenary yearbook of the British Goat Society.

to stand on the crest of the knoll, and I laid prone halfway down the hill, the goat's majestic outline would be accentuated against the sky. So far, so good. Billy was led out and set up in position. I lay flat, digging my elbows into the turf to hold the camera steady. I focused and framed the shot. The plan was that at a word from me, the owner would release his hold on Billy and step back out of the composition as I pressed the shutter. It was at that point that things went awry.

For some unknown reason Billy had taken an instant dislike to me. The moment Billy was released from restraint, he reared up on his hind legs, pivoted through ninety degrees and charged at me. The majestic figure on the skyline had transformed himself into a large and rapidly accelerating demon intent on attacking my person.

The self-preservation instinct, fuelled by adrenalin, is strong. I rolled from prone to upright in a fraction of a second and ran. It must have been a hilarious sight. I was being chased by a large, angry billy goat, who, in turn, was being chased by the farmer who was trying to regain control. Even more hilarious, the whole procedure was repeated a couple of dozen times in the course of the evening. Success depended on my ability to click the shutter between the release of Billy and my tactical retreat.

Billy was my one and only encounter with a malevolent goat, for they are generally the most gentle, sociable, and endearing of creatures.

Goats were introduced to this country by settlers in pre-Roman times and were the main source of milk supply. For hundreds of years there was no coherent planning in British goat breeding, but over the centuries a distinct type had emerged,

generally referred to as the Old English. Between 1850 and 1870 enlightened stockmen improved the milk yields of the breed, but by the mid twentieth century the breed was extinct in this country.

However, it did survive elsewhere.

Since Tudor times goats had been kept on board ship to provide milk and meat. Captain Cook must have kept appreciable numbers on his ships, for it was his habit to put ashore a few animals on remote islands to breed. Thus there would be a known and abundant source of milk and meat for ships passing that way. Between 1768 and 1799 he established several feral goat colonies in Australasia

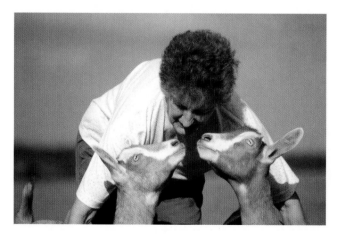

Goats can be very affectionate . . .

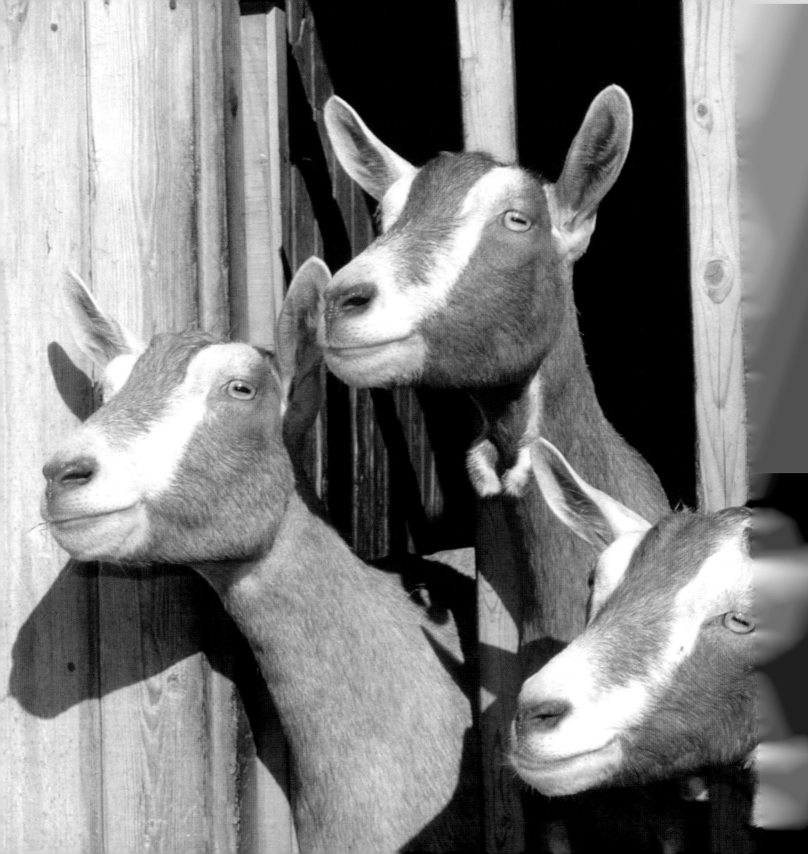

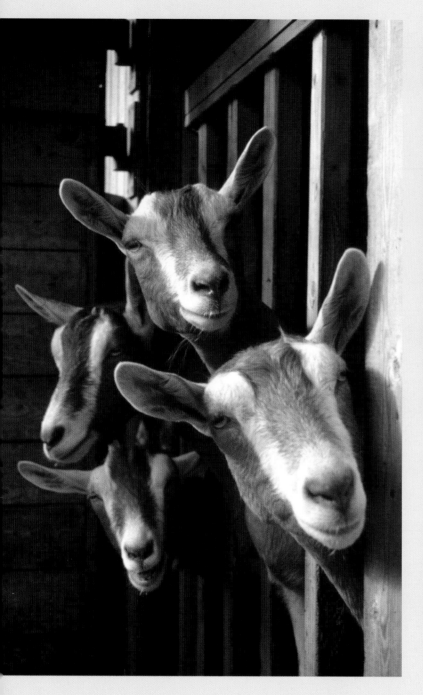
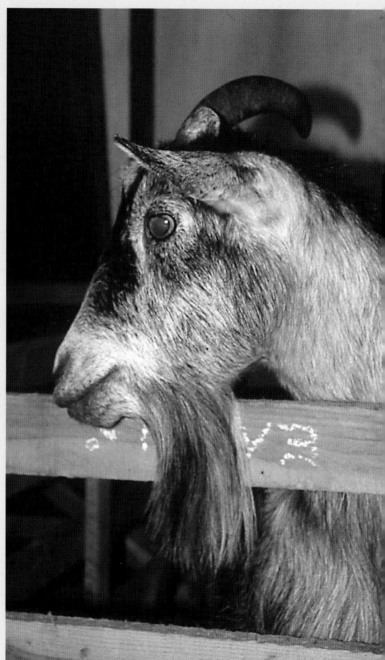

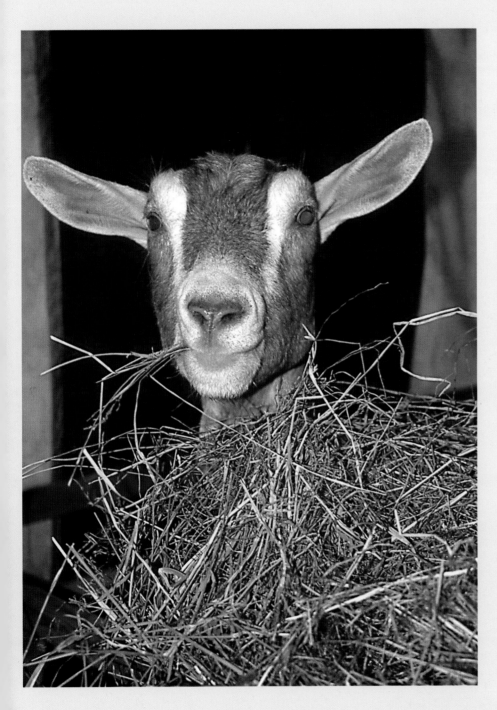

. . . and are great characters.

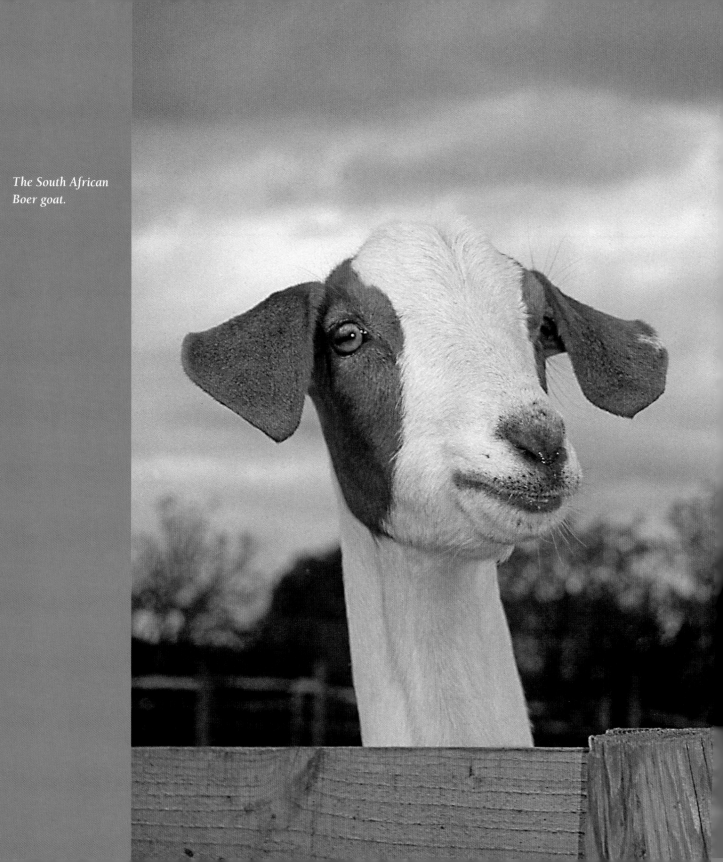

The South African Boer goat.

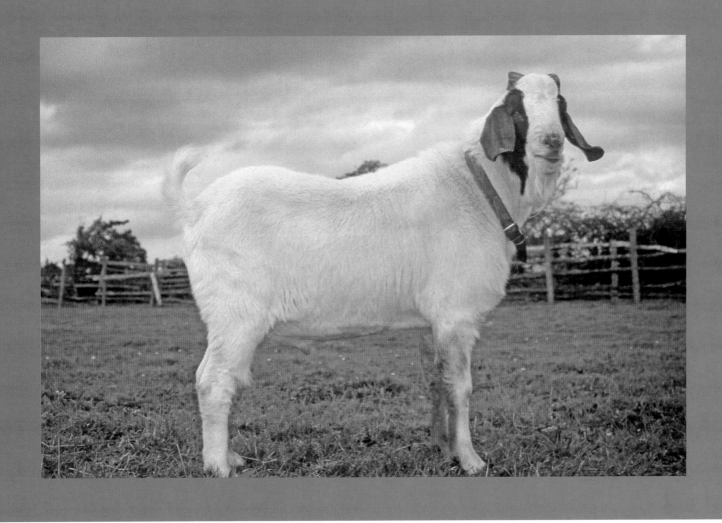

and the Pacific. Descendants of some of his goats that were put ashore on the island of Arapawa near New Zealand became so numerous that they had to be severely culled. Arapawa had become a living museum of the Old English breed.

The ship-board goat provided sustenance for passengers and crews throughout the Victorian era. The British Empire was then at its height and there was busy sea traffic from India, Africa, and the Mediterranean. As a result, hundreds of goats arriving from these countries ended up in zoos, parks, and even in the gardens and estates of retired colonial officers.

Cross-breeding of these animals was to result in the cosmopolitan nature of today's goat population.

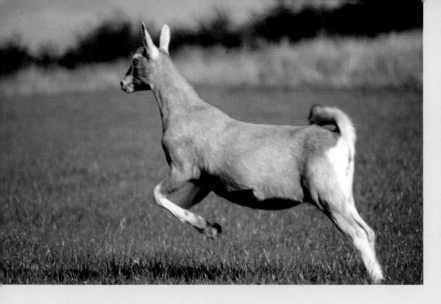

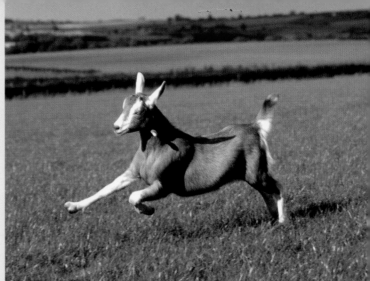

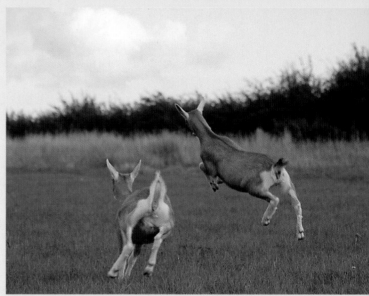

Goat enthusiasts further contributed to this trend by importing Swiss breeds with exceptional milking qualities.

In my professional life it's been a pleasure to meet and treat these characters, with the noted exception of Billy!

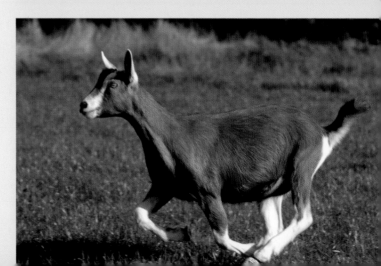

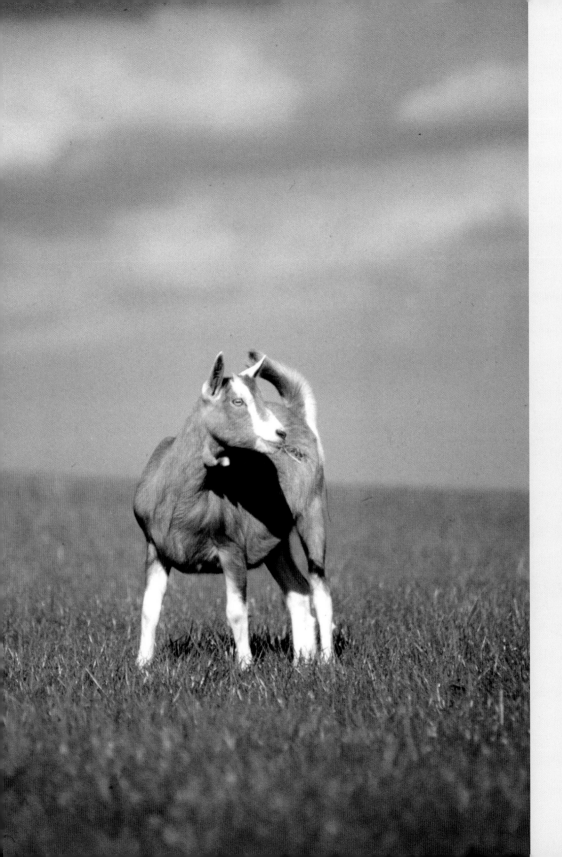

There's an expression, "full of the joys of spring". These youngsters are.

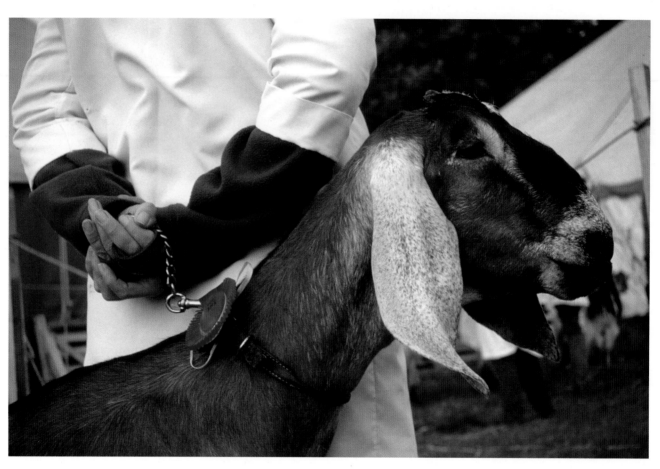

The British goat population is very cosmopolitan. In the days when sailing ships travelled the British Empire, goats were brought back from all corners of the world. This is an Anglo-Nubian.

13 Look What the Cat Brought In

I woke with a start and glanced at the clock. Four-thirty am. Something had roused me from a deep sleep. The early light of a summer dawn filtered through the bedroom window and I lay wondering what had disturbed me.

Then I heard it.

The sound from downstairs suggested that someone was ransacking the house. My pulse rate quickened and my mind was racing.

"What was that?" said my wife, Chris. "You'd better go and see what's going on."

Now I'm no hero, and the thought of confronting a burglar who may or may not have had an offensive weapon about his person did not appeal. However, I could not just lie there with mind and pulse in overdrive and do nothing.

I left my bed as noisily as possible and hit every light switch on my nerve-wracking way down the stairs. Surely the burglar would flee when he heard the occupant on his way to confrontation. I suppose that I should have put two and two together when I heard the cat flap rattle, but as I walked into the kitchen and switched on the light, there, parading around the kitchen floor, was a fully-grown woodcock. Was I dreaming?

I picked up the bird. Wings, legs, and plumage were all intact. There were a few ruffled feathers on the scruff of the neck, but I saw no good reason to defer his release. His strong flight into

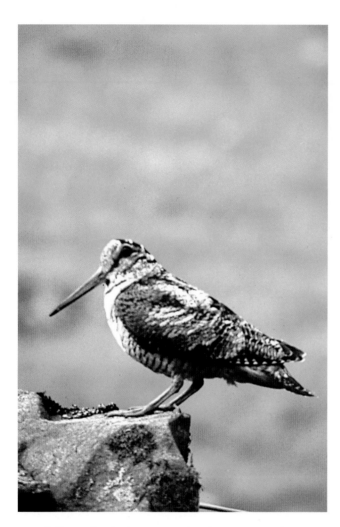

An adult woodcock, fourteen inches long. Our cat hauled one of these unceremoniously through our cat flap. No damage was done to either the bird or the cat flap!

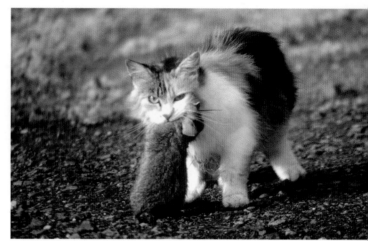

I spotted this cat returning from a hunting trip when I drove into a farmyard.

the woods at the bottom of the garden confirmed my appraisal of his condition. Only his dignity had been damaged.

Our cat burglar had, indeed, been our cat.

According to the *Hamlyn Guide to the Birds of Britain and Europe*, the length of the woodcock is fourteen inches, a third of which is made up of a long rigid beak. Chester, an avid hunter, had succeeded in manhandling this unfortunate fourteen-inch bird through a cat flap scarcely seven inches square. No wonder that the sounds of the night had suggested the house was being ransacked.

As might be expected from someone in my profession, I love to have cats and dogs as a part of the family. However, like most cat owners I deplore the fact that hunting and killing natural prey is often, although not always, a part of the cat's character. Whilst Chester was an avid hunter, his companion, Ritz, had no hunting instinct at all.

Because the domestic cat has been subjected to much less selective breeding than the dog, the physical and psychological characteristics of its wild ancestor often remain intact. Thus its predatory skills—stalking, chasing, catching, and killing—are often equal to those of the African wildcat from which it is descended. Whilst most cat owners consider hunting deplorable, in the farmyard it is a distinct advantage. Not only is the cat a pleasant creature to have on the farm, but it is a low-maintenance, highly efficient rodent controller.

Cats' hearing is phenomenal, probably having the power to detect a greater range of frequencies than any other mammal. It is particularly sensitive at high frequencies, which correspond to the high-pitched squeaking of mice and rats. In addition to this, each of the wide, trumpet-shaped external ears can be moved independently to aid direction-finding of sound sources.

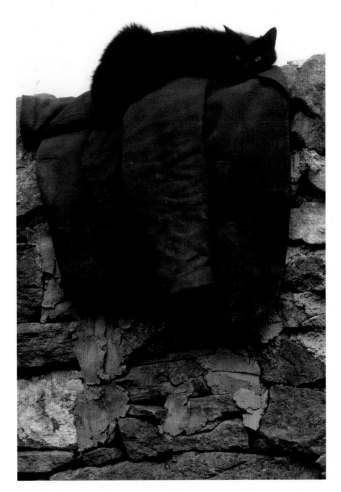

A comfortable seat on a farmer's jacket on a wall . . .

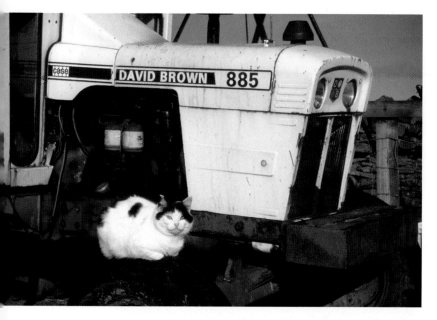

. . . and on a tractor wheel . . .

The eyes, too, are remarkable and are well adapted to night vision. The large eyes, set squarely at the front of the skull, give a wide angle of sight and the pupils can dilate markedly.

These physical adaptations to a predatory lifestyle accompany the hunting instinct. Although it would seem logical to assume that a well-fed cat would have a reduced motivation to hunt, this is not so. It appears that even generous feeding will not reduce hunting.

To quote Valerie O'Farrell and Peter Neville from their *Manual of Feline Behaviour*:

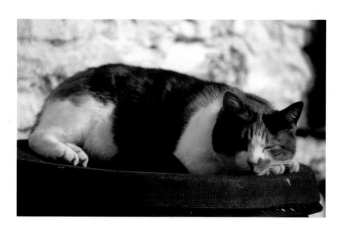

. . . and on a dustbin lid . . .

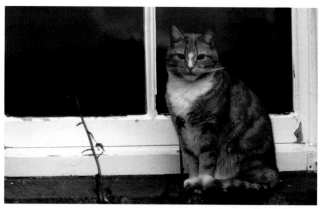

. . . and on a windowsill.

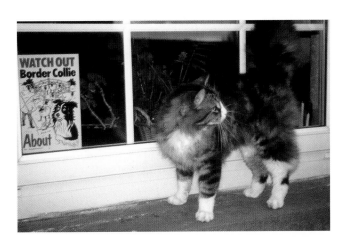

The notice reads, "Watch out, Border Collie about." This cat looks as though he's just spotted it.

" If they have the opportunity most cats will hunt and kill small animals, some being more enthusiastic and skilful hunters than others.

Although most owners are philosophical and learn to live with this aspect of cats' behavioural repertoire some are upset by it. It may be of some comfort to them to reflect that cats evolved into predators over millions of years, long before they were domesticated. "

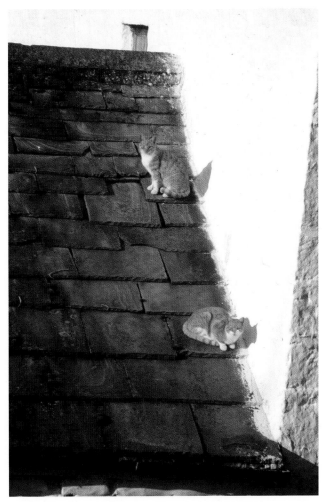

These two look as though they are just relaxing on the roof, but always there is the hunting instinct. They were actually trying to catch newly fledged swallows. I'm pleased to report that they had no success.

The classic cat up a tree.
I don't think this will need
to be rescued by the fire
brigade!

14 A Dog's Chance of Happiness

It was Mark Twain who wrote, "If you pick up a starving dog and make him prosperous he will not bite you. This is the principal difference between a dog and a man."

That's quite a sweeping statement, but it's so true. Once you have earned the love and respect of a dog, it is unconditional, and it is enduring. Nothing will shake it.

Sadly there are many who acquire a dog on a whim, without any thought of the commitment necessary for responsible ownership. The novelty soon wears off and the poor pup, having spent the first few precious months of his life in a dysfunctional relationship, ends up at the rescue kennels if he's lucky. Many are simply abandoned. The rescue

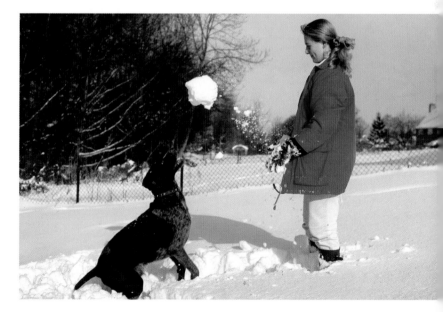

Our daughter, Laura, playing snowballs with Rye in our garden.

organisations do wonderful work. Everyone has heard of the Battersea Dogs' Home, and many have heard of the National Canine Defence League, but there are also scores of local charities that work hard to home waifs and strays.

Almost all of my colleagues and our office staff owned dogs, and a good proportion of these were rescued from the scrap heap. Paul met Judy as a pup with a shattered leg after a road accident. The owner didn't want to know about the expense and bother of saving her life. With dedication and a high degree of orthopaedic skill, Paul remodelled the leg, and Judy became his constant companion for more than ten years.

Pat, one of our veterinary nurses, took pity on a failed sheepdog pup destined for euthanasia. She adopted him, took him to obedience classes, and turned Shep into a winner at Crufts. This doomed pup changed Pat's life, for following numerous Crufts wins, she forged a successful career as an internationally renowned dog trainer.

I have been a dog owner for about twenty-five years, always acquiring a rescue dog: one that "needs a good home". In that time I have owned German Pointers, and have experienced the joys, frustrations, and responsibilities of pet ownership. I have also, inevitably, experienced the sadness and the grief that comes at the end of a happy partnership.

Blue was a crazy one-year-old when I met him in a temporary home on a farm. He had spent his first year in a flat in Newcastle, a totally unsuitable environment for this exuberant, energetic, athletic breed. His frustration had left its mark on most of the furniture and doors of his original home, and he had to go. He was totally undisciplined and unmanageable. He didn't even know the word "sit". In his first week with us he managed to devour the Sunday joint (before it was cooked), a bar of soap, some of my post mortem specimens, and most of the interior of my car. A visit to a local scrapyard to purchase the whole of the interior of a Renault 4 did nothing to further our relationship.

But help was at hand. Ken Saxby, our village policeman, came to the rescue. Ken was a wise and knowledgeable man who had had extensive experience as a dog handler in the police force. He was so generous with his time and patience, not only training my new and delinquent charge, but also training me how to handle a dog; how to think like a dog.

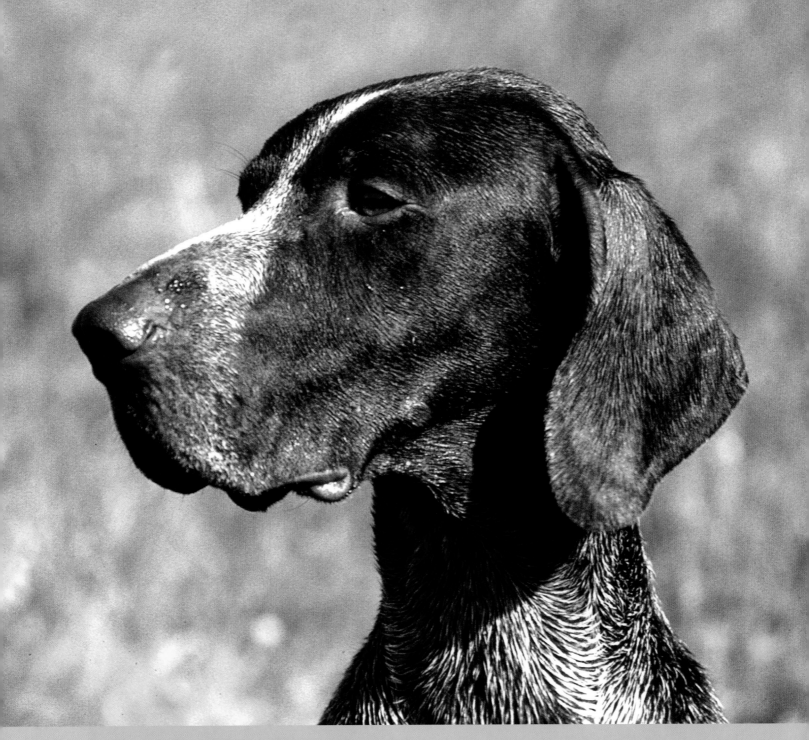

Blue joined our family as a delinquent one-year-old who destroyed the interior of my car. With some expert advice I was able to break all his bad habits and he became my constant companion for thirteen years.

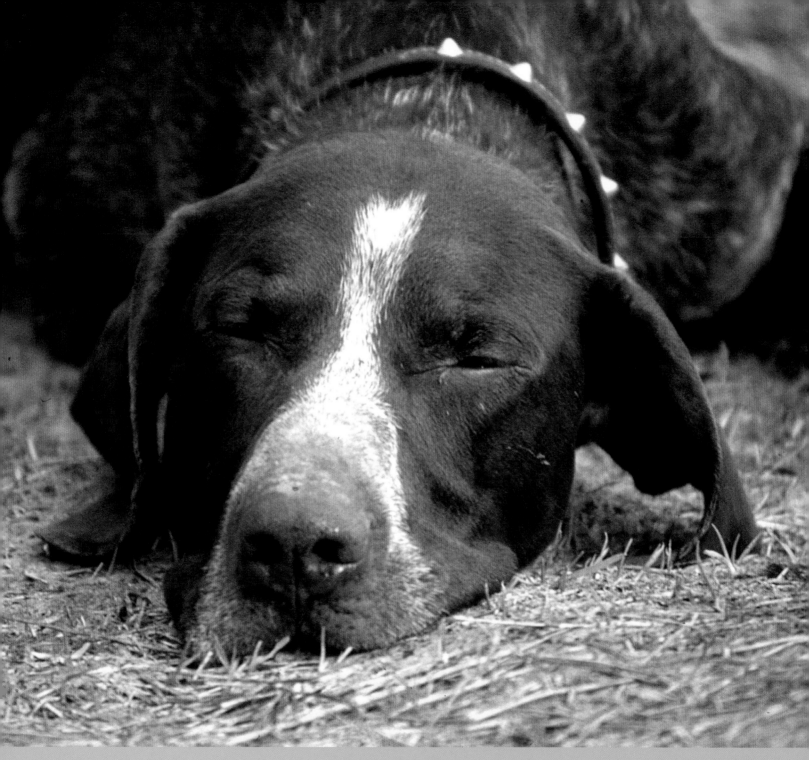

Blue taking a nap.

Within a few weeks Blue's discipline was impeccable. He would respond to voice commands, whistles, and hand signals. Even when he was three hundred yards away a blast from my whistle would stop him in his tracks and he'd sit. We became inseparable. When the phone rang in the middle of the night he would take up a position by the back door, knowing that I was going out on a call and letting me know that I mustn't forget to take him with me.

Our parting was sad, but it did much to help me to understand at first hand the heavy decision that many pet owners eventually have to make. Blue had reached the ripe old age of fourteen, and had struggled for some time with chronic illness. Gradually the treatment was becoming less effective. At five o'clock one morning, after we had both spent a sleepless night, I knew that he had had enough. He lay trustingly with his head on my lap as I did what had to be done.

It took some time to get over that loss. It was tempting to dash out and buy another dog immediately, but I resisted the temptation. Instead I let it be known that if anyone knew of a German Pointer needing a good home, I'd be interested. Eventually I heard of a three-year-old whose owner

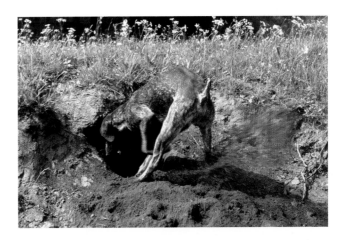

Blue loved digging into rabbit holes . . .

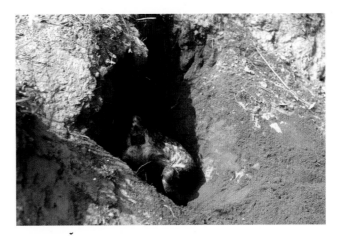

. . . until he was almost out of sight. He never ever caught a rabbit.

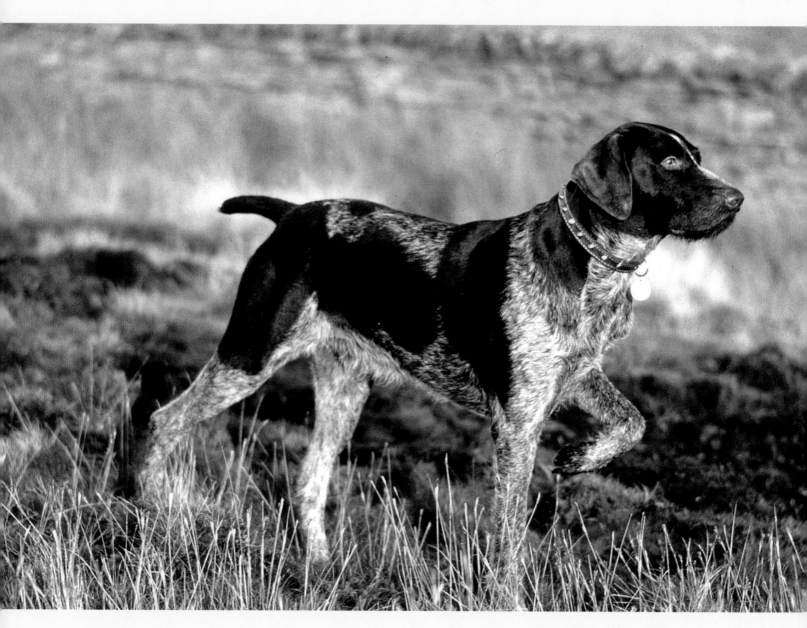

Blue's successor was Rye, another German Pointer, and a great character. At the scent of game he would freeze in the classic pointing pose.

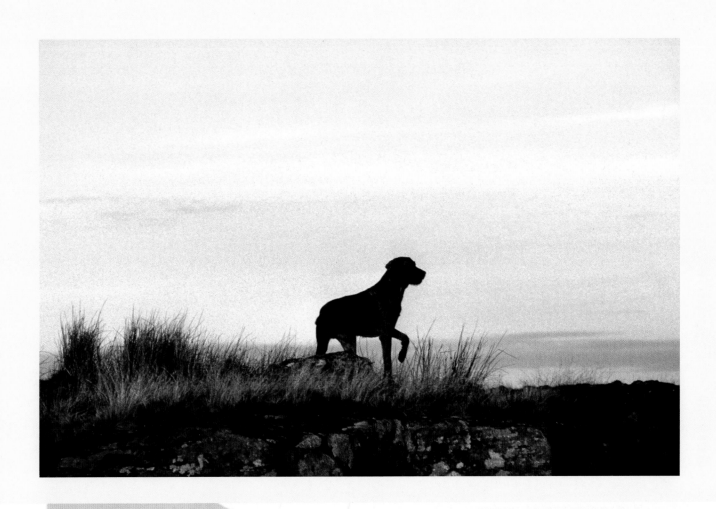

had died tragically. There would never be another Blue, but Rye, too, was something special.

His late owner had been the most diligent of dog owners. She had taken Rye to obedience classes and developed his great sense of fun. Sit, stay, recall, and walking to heel were all carried out to perfection.

Often I didn't need to give the command. Rye knew exactly what was required.

His instinctive pointing skills were brilliant. A walk in the country was punctuated by the dog freezing in the classic pointing position, immobile and with a foreleg raised. When that happened you could be

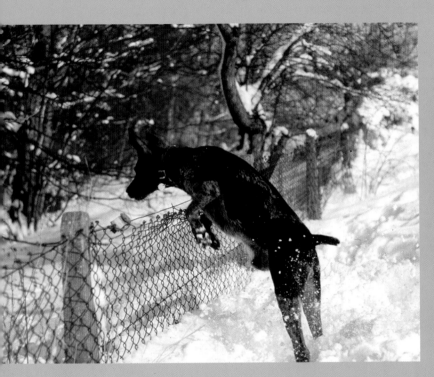

Rye was eager to learn, and I taught him the command "over", at which he would jump over the fence. I took lots of action shots of his athletic leaps, and was there when he didn't quite make it. His feet slipped and he crashed into the fence. The only harm done was to his dignity!

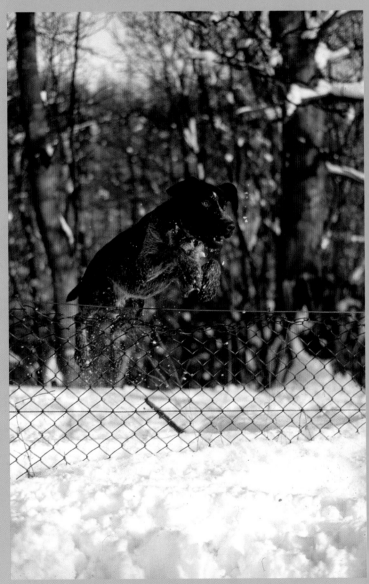

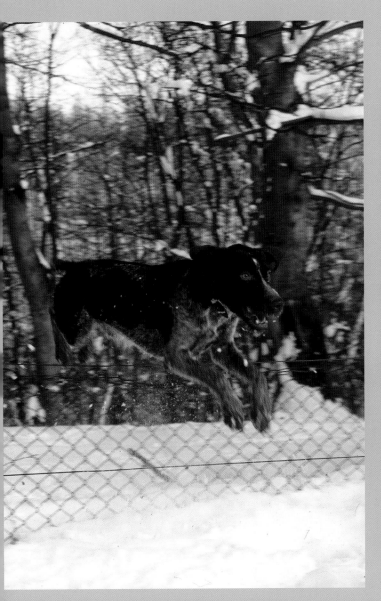
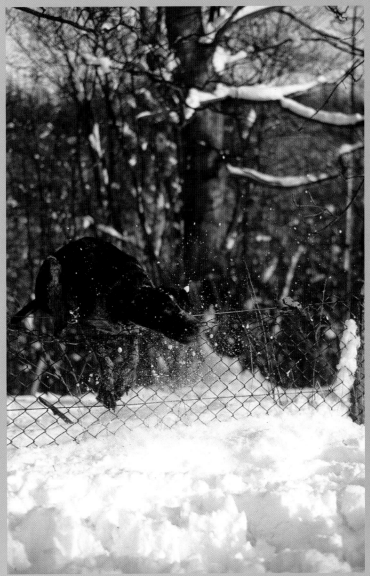

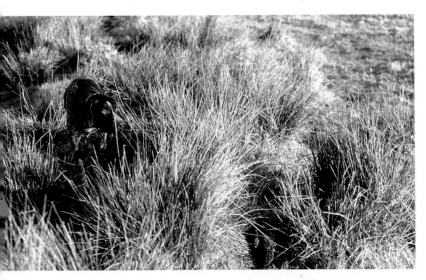

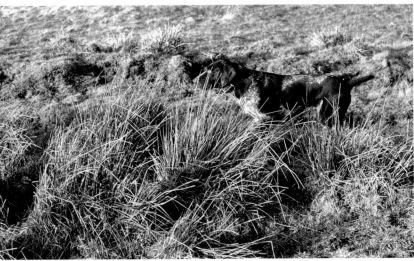

A remarkable scenario. Rye pointing a pheasant with both dog and bird locked in immobility.

sure that there was a rabbit or pheasant somewhere in a straight line upwind of his nose. I'm not into shooting, but these gundog skills were a thrill to see. On one occasion he froze, and, most unusually, I could see dog and pheasant. Neither was going to move, and I circled the scenario, shooting a whole roll of film as a record of this amazing sight.

Teaching him new commands was a delight, for he took part with eagerness. I taught him the command "over" in minutes. The dog is put in the sitting position next to a fence or a wall on the opposite side to the owner. There he will stay till the command is given. "Over" probably is construed as a recall and the dog leaps the fence to join his master. Eventually the dog can be persuaded to make the leap away or towards the owner. All these lessons were treated as games by Rye, and it was such fun. It was also a great opportunity to take pictures of him sailing over, a foot clear of the fence.

With a mixture of telepathy and subtle hand signals, I could put him through his paces without giving any obvious commands. Once when we had some French visitors, I couldn't resist telling them that Rye understood French. I executed retrieves, deliveries, and walking to heel as well as the basic sit, stay, and recall, all with voice commands in

French. They were amazed. To this day I think they believed that Rye was fluent in French!

And as a parting shot I informed them that he spoke German too!

I do hope that the moral of my tale is self-evident. There is great fun and satisfaction in responsible pet ownership. If you do decide to acquire a dog, consider the rescue associations. Any vet will point you in the right direction, or may even know of a suitable animal himself. If discipline is a problem, go along to obedience classes where you and your dog will be trained.

And with a bit of luck you'll have years of experiencing the joy of having a happy, healthy devoted dog as part of the family.

15 Lambing Time

Easter wouldn't be Easter without fluffy chicks in the farmyard, a "host of golden daffodils", and fields full of lambs skipping about in the spring sunshine. However, it's pretty tough being a lamb, and the problems start even before you're born.

If Mum hasn't succumbed to any of half a dozen infections that result in abortion or stillbirth, she could yet be affected by metabolic diseases such as Staggers or Twin Lamb Disease. The former is a rapidly fatal drop in blood calcium levels, although prompt treatment by the shepherd will avert disaster. The latter is an insidious form of pregnancy toxaemia, which is much less responsive to treatment.

Low copper levels in the ewe's blood during pregnancy will lead to abnormal development of the lamb's nervous system, resulting in an incurable cerebral palsy-like condition called Swayback.

And so the lamb is born—but that's not the end of the story. For the first few days of life the little fellow faces a harrowing set of challenges. Some ewes at this stage get fed up with the whole business and reject the lamb, physically butting him whenever he approaches. Other ewes may be motherly but fail to produce milk for the first day or two. Hypothermia and starvation may ensue.

The lamb's wet navel immediately after birth provides an excellent medium for entry of all manner of germs which can cause peritonitis, liver abscesses, and septic arthritis. Various viruses and bacteria can cause acute diarrhoea or toxaemia.

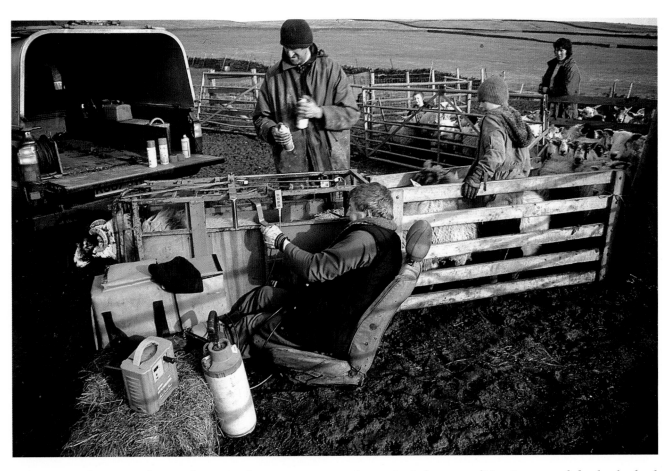

It doesn't seem long since ultrasound scanning for pregnancy was an innovation in human medicine. It says much for the shepherd that he was quick to adopt the technique for his flock. In this picture the sheep are herded through a race into a holding crate.

And so, when you see those happy bands of healthy lambs gambolling across the fields in the spring sunshine, spare a thought for the flockmaster who has carefully monitored the ewe's condition throughout the previous summer and the five-month pregnancy. The ewe will probably have been

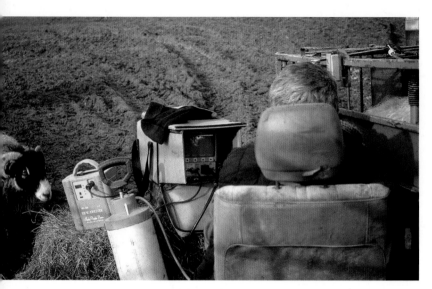

The scanning operative sits in a low seat, runs the probe over the sheep's abdomen and watches the screen in front of him.

Clostridial diseases, not only protecting the dam, but passing on maternal antibodies to the lamb via the first rich milk, termed "colostrum". In many cases the ewes are housed before, during, and for the first few days after lambing. This provides warm, clean, dry surroundings for the delivery, and establishment of the bond between ewe and lamb.

scanned to identify single and multiple pregnancies so that those carrying twins and triplets can have special feeding. It doesn't seem so long since ultrasound scans were introduced to human medicine, but the shepherds were quick to realise its usefulness in flock management.

The ewe may have been injected with a copper supplement to avoid Swayback. Almost every ewe has completed a vaccination course against deadly

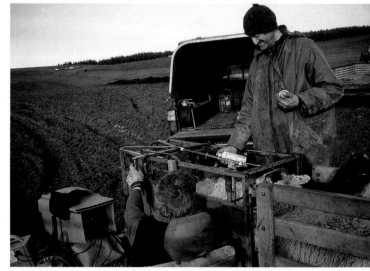

The farmer stands by with coloured marking aerosols to record the result of the scan. A combination of colour marks will indicate whether or not the ewe is pregnant, or how many lambs she is carrying. Her feeding regime can then be adjusted accordingly.

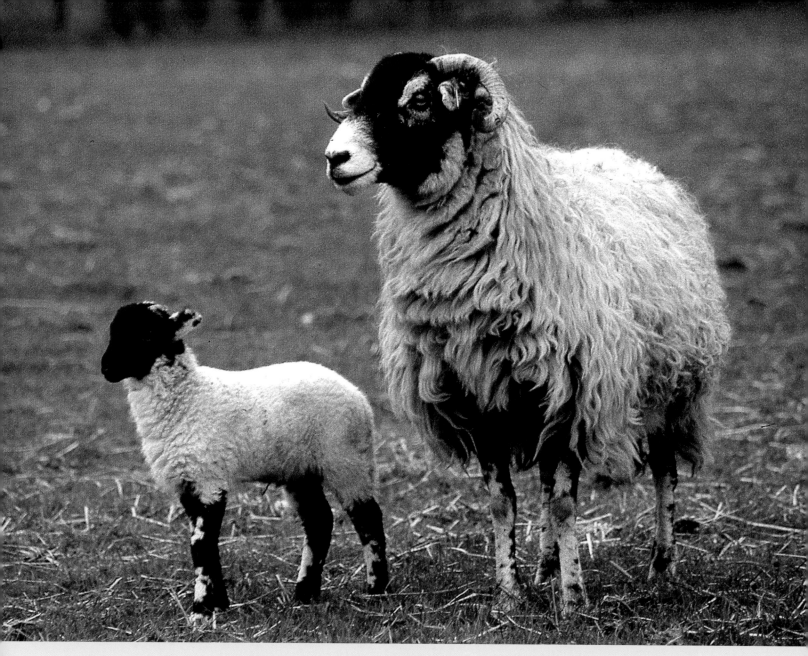

A Swaledale ewe usually has a single lamb.

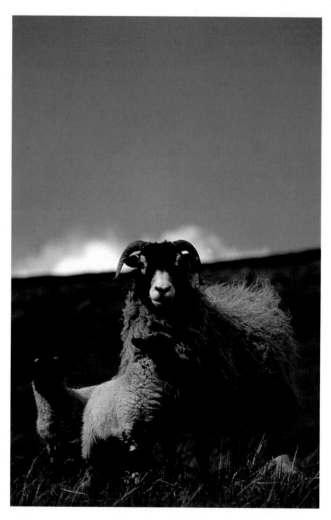

Occasionally they will produce twins.

Navels are soaked in antiseptic at birth. The shepherd then checks each ewe's milk supply and the lamb's ability to feed. Most shepherds are expert at passing a stomach tube to feed a weakly lamb.

And so, like most things in life, there's more to lambing time than meets the eye. Behind every successful healthy lamb crop there's a wealth of dedication and technological expertise.

The next time you stop to admire a field full of contented ewes and gambolling lambs, by all means marvel at the wonders of nature, but I suggest you take your hat off to the shepherd whose skill and dedication has made it possible.

Most shepherds are accomplished at delivering lambs. In fact there were certain farms where we knew that if we were called to a delivery, it would be a very difficult one. We were also aware of the problems associated with each breed.

On farms where there were pedigree Swaledales, we often had challenging cases. The Swaledale ewe's pelvis is quite narrow, making it quite difficult to manipulate the presentation of the lamb. Add to this the fact that many male lambs are born with well-developed horn buds. Having one's fingers

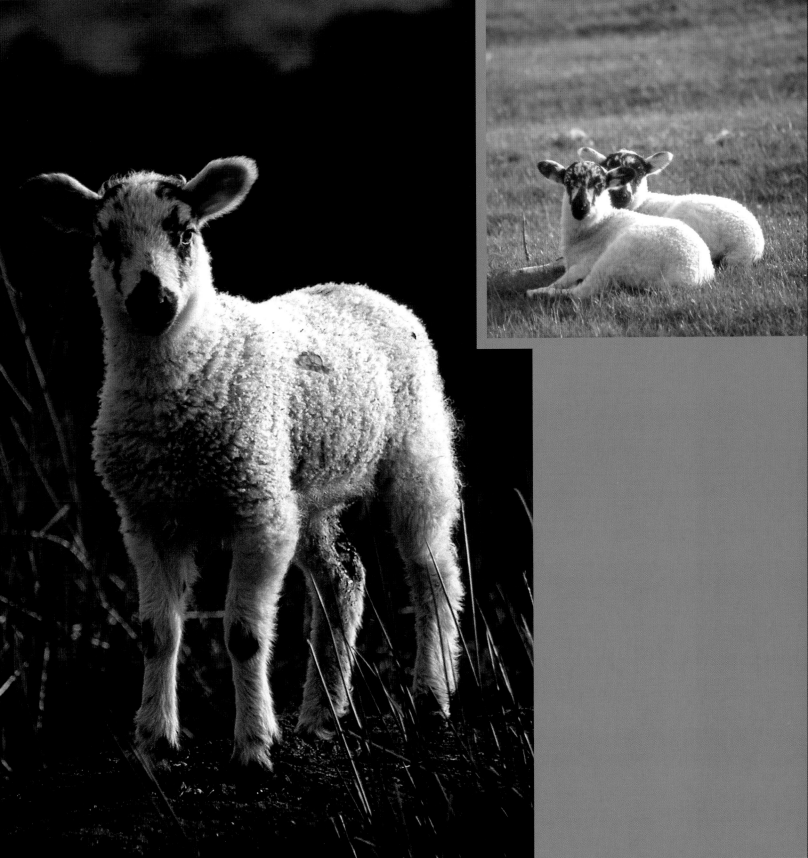

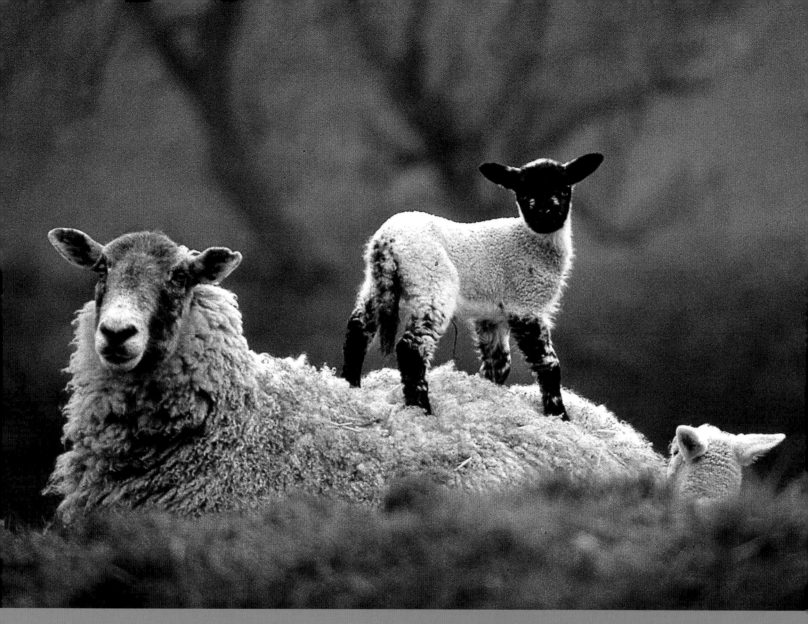

You have to be really quick to capture this picture. When the ewe sees you approach, she will stand up and the lamb will fall off.

jammed between a tup lamb's head and the dam's pelvis can bring tears to the eyes!

Another painful memory is delivering Texel lambs. The Texel ewe is a much bigger animal than the Swaledale, but, again, the pelvis is narrow. Whilst horns are not a problem here, the lamb has a very broad forehead. Using one's hand as a "shoehorn" to ease the head through the pelvis at delivery can be every bit as excruciating as a Swaledale case.

There is a condition referred to as "ringwomb" by the shepherds. This is where lambing should be happening, but the cervix fails to dilate and there is not room for the lamb to pass through the birth canal. In most cases where we were called to this condition, lots of lubricant and patience, coupled with gentle manual dilation of the cervix, was successful. Very occasionally these efforts met with no success, and as any delay would result in stillbirth, the only alternative was to perform a caesarean section.

On one memorable occasion I was called to a pedigree Leicester ewe with ringwomb and performed a caesarean in the middle of a field. It seemed easier to do it there, so I drove my car across to her. The farmer brought hot water, soap, and a towel.

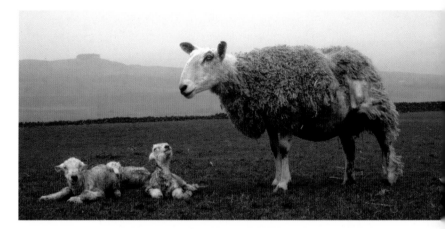

This picture was taken immediately after I had performed a caesarean section on a Leicester ewe.

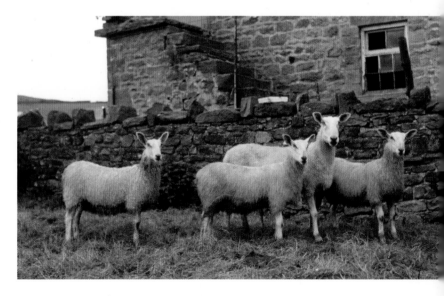

This is the same family three months later.

It was a beautiful spring day. The sun was shining; the birds were singing; the operation went like clockwork. Since the surgery was performed under local anaesthetic, the ewe was able to attend to her three strong, healthy pedigree lambs immediately. Mother and babies progressed well. It was such a lovely sight that I took a picture of the scene.

Three months later I was on the same farm, and when I had completed my task, the farmer asked if I'd like to see the Leicester ewe and her offspring. They had done really well, so again I reached for my camera. Stage-managing four sheep for the camera is near impossible but eventually we managed it.

Comparing the two pictures sums up what a privilege it is to be a veterinary surgeon.

16 Horsepower and Heritage

I'm immensely proud of my profession and its ability to care for "all creatures great and small", but it wasn't always so. It was in 1785 that the Odiham Agricultural Society held a meeting which produced a resolution to promote the study of farriery upon rational scientific principles. Six years later their deliberations resulted in the establishment of the Royal Veterinary College in London.

For 150 years the profession was centred on the horse, in both military and civilian roles. Farm animals were treated by the old "cow doctors", who had lots of experience but no scientific training. It wasn't till a government report in 1938 suggesting vets should study farm animals that things started to change.

Even when I was at veterinary college in Edinburgh in the 1960s, we spent a whole year studying the anatomy of the horse. And yet a whole generation of vets hardly saw a horse, between its demise as a working animal and its resurrection in recreation and sport.

Scarcely more than a century ago horsepower actually meant working with horses. It was only in 1903 that Henry Ford launched the Ford Motor Company, and not until 1913 that he installed the first mass production line. Steam trains had been around since the 1840s, but unless you had ready access to the fledgling rail network, you were still totally dependant on the horse.

In the dales, a popular breed of pony was the strong and hardy Scottish Galloway from the south-west

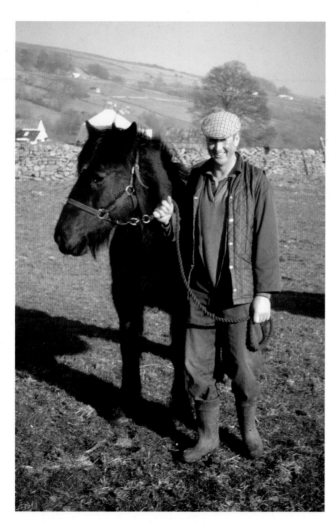

of Scotland. Many were brought to the Pennines in the seventeenth century where they interbred with local stock to give the forerunner of the Dales Pony. Some Clydesdale blood was introduced to increase size and strength. Norfolk Trotter and Yorkshire Roadster blood was added to give a sure-footed, high-stepping gait not unlike the Hackney. A Welsh Cob stallion, "Comet", also added his stamp to the breed.

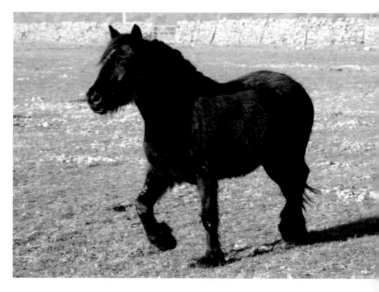

Richie Longstaff is a knowledgeable Dales Pony breeder. His father, along with a few enthusiasts, did much to save the breed from extinction in the 1950s.

The Dales Pony has powerful hindquarters and a sure-footed, high-stepping gait.

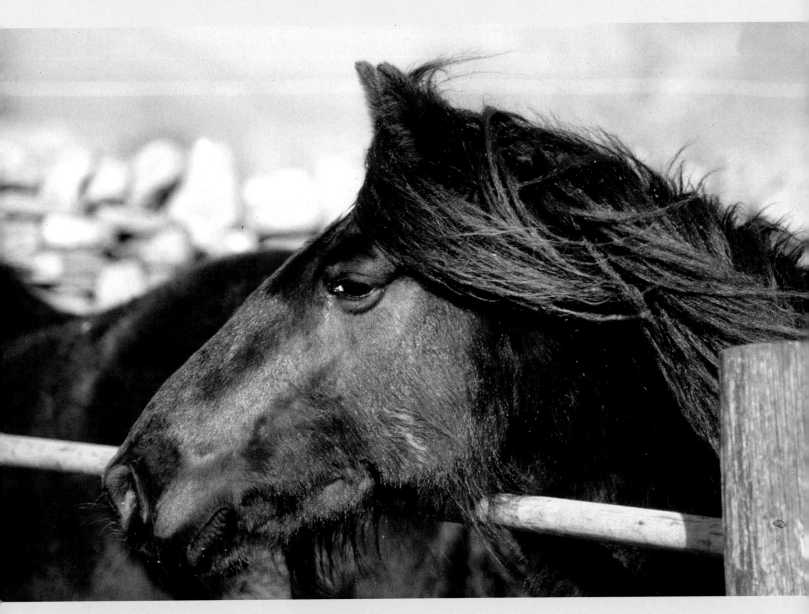

Perhaps most importantly it has a kind face and biddable temperament.

In the meantime the Scottish Galloway Pony became extinct.

Throughout this breeding programme the Dales Pony retained its basic character of being hardy, strong, and biddable. Not only was it of use in the lead industry, but it became the basic power unit on most dales farms. Under the saddle it was the ideal shepherd's pony, and between the shafts it could pull a cart or a sledge carrying a ton. Its quiet nature made it a joy to work with.

In the early years of the twentieth century there was commercial demand for heavier animals, and many owners were only too ready to cross their mares with Clydesdale stallions. Fortunately there were also owners who saw this threat to the pure breed. In order to preserve the integrity of the type, they formed the "Dales Pony Improvement Society" and opened a stud book in 1916.

The modern Dales Pony Society breed standard states, "A Dales Pony should move with a great deal of energy and power, lifting their hooves well clear of the ground. The overall impression should be of an alert, courageous, but calm and kind animal."

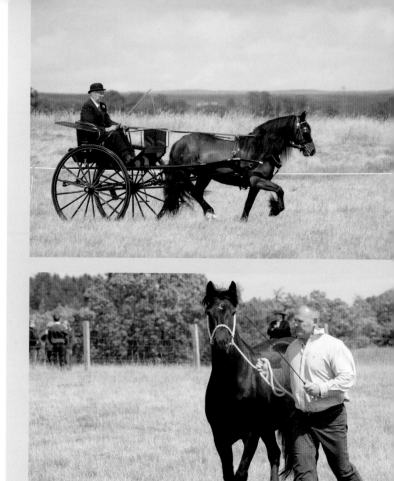

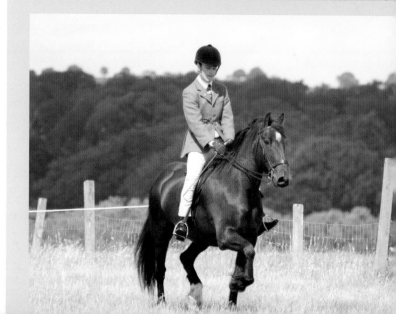

The Dales Pony is an elegant mover in hand, between the shafts, and under the saddle.

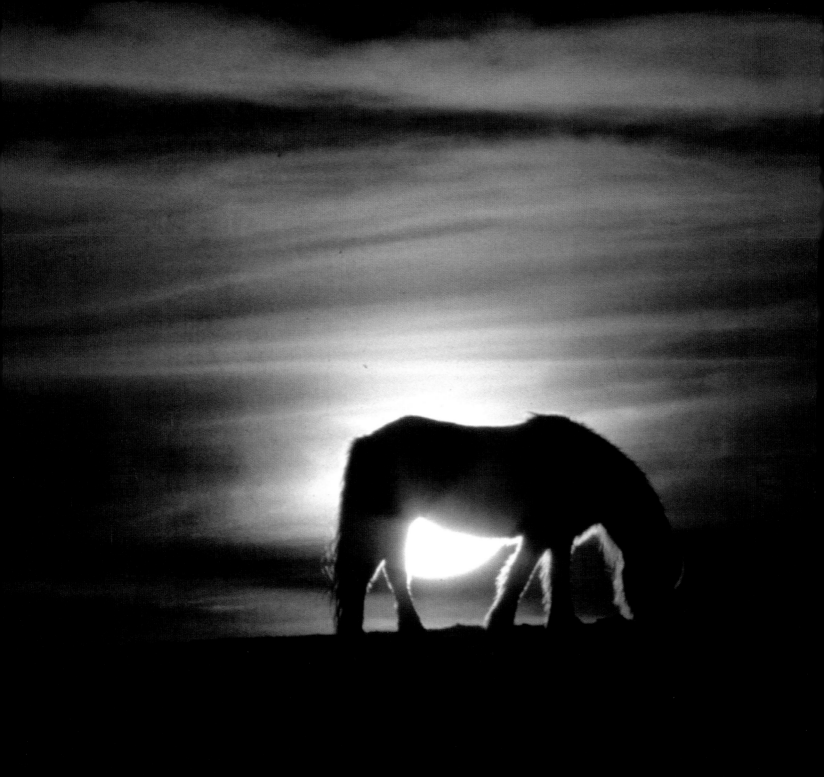

Thousands of these useful animals were conscripted in two world wars, never to return. Dales Ponies became scarce in their native dales, for in the post-war world of agriculture the tractor had arrived. The role of the Dales Pony as the basic power unit of the Pennines was over.

By the 1950s the breed was on the brink of extinction, and had it not been for a handful of dedicated enthusiasts, it would have disappeared altogether. They sought as many ponies as they could that exhibited the typical Dales conformation and temperament.

Teesdale still has a dedicated band of knowledgeable enthusiasts who numbered amongst our clients, so I was privileged to become familiar with this animal that is so much a part of our dales heritage.

In its centenary year I wish the Dales Pony Society continued success in ensuring the endurance of a very special breed.

A Dales Pony at sunset.

17 Things They Never Told You at College

Back in the sixties, veterinary education centred on the anatomy of the horse, the cow, the dog, and the "fowl". Physiology concentrated in depth on the functions of the four stomachs of sheep and cows. I left college in 1968, secure in the knowledge that whatever general practice threw at me, I'd have a good grasp of what it took to make a pretty competent diagnosis. Horses, cattle, sheep, pigs, dogs, cats, and the common domestic pets had been studied until we knew almost everything that could possibly go wrong with them.

No one had ever thought that one day we may have opened the consulting room door and called, "Next please", to be confronted by a salamander.

(A colleague of mine working in South Yorkshire once had to deal with a sick, fourteen-foot-long python. Its owner was an "exotic dancer" who used the snake as part of her act.)

However, back to the salamander. He was an amazing little creature. His basic shape was that of a large lizard. He looked as though he'd been moulded in glossy black plastic, and had iridescent yellow blotches here and there on his body. He was beautiful. But his toes were falling off! After a cursory examination I made a feeble excuse and retired to the office to consult my colleagues.

"Does anyone know anything about salamanders?" I pleaded.

None of my colleagues did. But serendipity, a favourite friend in tight situations, came up trumps again.

There happened to be, in the office, at that very time, a rep from a drug company.

"My boss is an authority on salamanders," he said. "Why don't you give him a call?"

I couldn't believe my good fortune. I made the call, discussed the symptoms with a very knowledgeable and sympathetic veterinary surgeon on the other end of the phone, and was able to make a positive diagnosis. I was also able to institute the necessary treatment. What a fantastic stroke of luck.

As I drove to my first encounter with an alpaca, I was possessed by a similar, although not so profound, insecurity. Camelids (the collective name for camels, llamas, vicunas, guanacos, and alpacas) were, after all, ruminants with a similar anatomy and physiology to cattle, sheep, and goats. And the problem was a basic one. An alpaca baby had been born with a jaw defect. It could not suckle. The solution was there in my little black bag. A stomach tube designed for lambs was used to fill the little one's stomach with precious colostrum and milk. "Sophie", as she was named, overcame her disability. Thanks to dedicated attention from her owners, she achieved adolescence, although her congenital abnormalities eventually precluded her survival to a ripe old age.

From that very first meeting I was so impressed by this relatively new species that had appeared on the "day-book" at the surgery. Alpacas are gentle and inquisitive creatures, each one with an individual character. They are so endearing, with big dark eyes peering through their dangling dreadlocks. You'd even say that they have a knowing smile and an impish sense of humour.

Six thousand years ago the native South Americans took the wild guanaco and domesticated the species to produce the beast of burden we now know as the llama. At the same time the wild vicuna was domesticated for its fine fleece, and the result was the alpaca. In the sixteenth and seventeenth century the Conquistadors wrought havoc in South America. They virtually destroyed the Incan civilisation, and with it, their fine herds of alpaca. It is only in recent decades that interest in the alpaca has been revived, and breeders strive to reproduce the fine qualities and genetic excellence that were obliterated by the Spanish invaders four centuries ago.

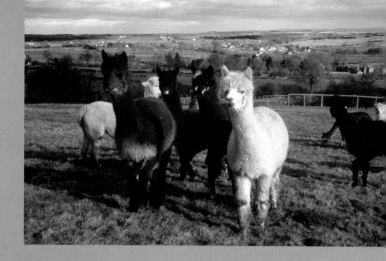

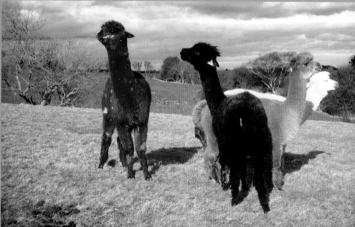

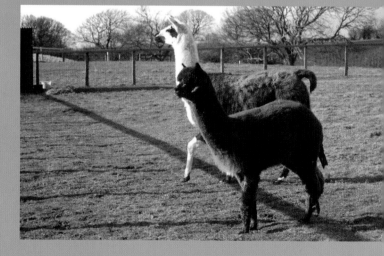

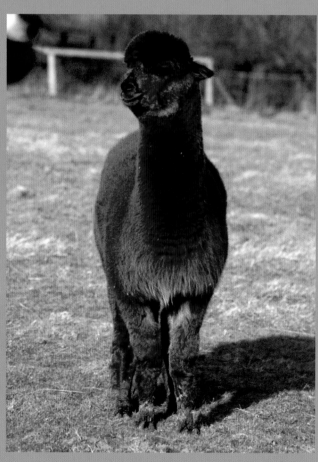

Alpacas.

Not only in South America, but also in North America, Australia, and in our country, people have rediscovered the species and its potential as a companion animal and a producer of the raw material for a luxurious fabric. There were, apparently, ten thousand alpaca in the UK in 2003. Recent estimates suggest that there could be many more today. Breeders are striving to reach herd numbers and fleece quality that would allow a viable large-scale industry in the UK, producing fabrics from home-produced wool.

Production of alpaca cloth in the UK is not a new idea. In 1836 Titus Salt first came upon alpaca wool from South America, and saw its huge potential. He made his fortune from manufacturing fabrics made from the wool. When alpaca dresses found favour with Queen Victoria, his already phenomenal success reached new heights. He became an extremely wealthy man and built new mills and a model village for his workers on a twenty-five-acre site in the Aire valley. The village of Saltaire is now a World Heritage Site, and it was founded on wealth generated from the alpaca.

Large-scale fabric manufacture from home-grown UK fibre is still a long way away. The reproduction rate of the alpaca is slow. Only one baby (known as a "cria") is produced each year. However, the alpaca seems to have adapted well from its home in the Andes to our temperate pastures. Dedicated and knowledgeable alpaca farmers are breeding towards top-quality stock that will produce the finest of fibres. Let us hope that they achieve success.

18 Oh for the Wings, for the Wings, of a . . . DUCK!

I n the whole of my career, I don't think I've seen anything as funny as a drunken duck. Pet ducks are regularly, though not frequently, presented as patients. When they do appear, the case is sure to be bemusing, challenging, and unusual.

The owner of the above-mentioned duck suspected that his pet had been poisoned. This was certainly a reasonable tentative diagnosis, as the patient waddled in a bizarre manner, falling over at regular intervals, and quacking dementedly. However, after asking a few questions, it transpired that the duck had had access to an orchard, and I suspected that he

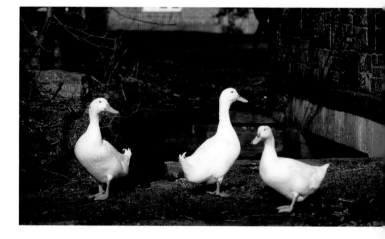

Ducks are the characters of the avian world. They seem to exude "attitude".

had been feeding on fermenting windfall apples—naturally occurring cider. He was admitted for a course of concentrated B vitamins to help the liver deal with its processing of an alcohol overload, and was discharged the next morning, a much subdued and sober character. It would appear that ducks can have hangovers too.

Another satisfying and successful case was that of a wild female mallard, brought to the surgery with a length of fishing line protruding from her mouth. An X-ray picture showed a fish hook embedded in the oesophagus. We operated to remove the offending object and hospitalised the patient till we were sure that she could feed and swallow well. It was a great feeling to release the duck on the riverbank where she had been found. She flew straight over to her companions, obviously delighted to be home.

Yet another duck patient was presented with serious damage to its ankle joint. There seemed very little that anyone could do and I began to break the news as gently as possible to the lady owner. When I saw tears welling up in her eyes I swiftly changed tack, and although I knew that the chances of success were incredibly slim, I fashioned a padded metal splint to hold the joint at its natural angle of

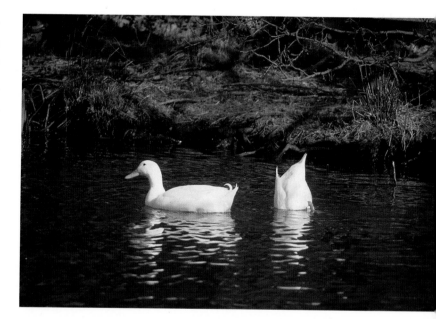

One and a half ducks.

ninety degrees. To cut a long story short, it worked. Youthful optimism rules OK!

There was, however, a particular duck of which I shall always retain a fond memory, and he even had a name.

We had just appointed a new assistant, Robert, and he was staying at our house until his flat near to the practice was ready. My wife, Chris, had prepared dinner at about seven-thirty, and at nine o'clock we

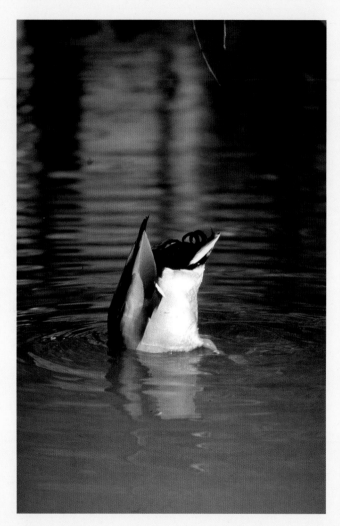

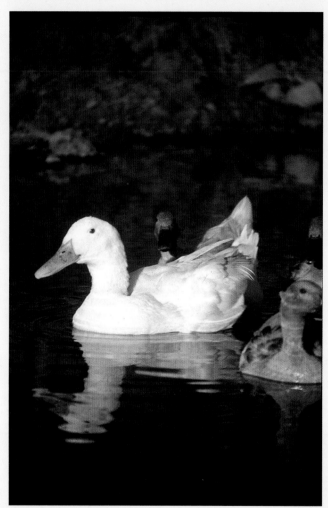

Half a duck.   *A portrait of Daffy.*

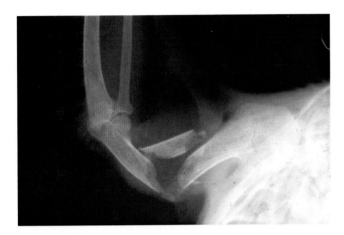

An X-ray of Daffy's wing revealed a shattered humerus in three distinct pieces.

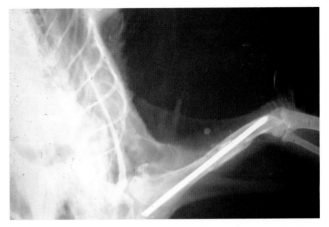

We asked Daffy's owner to bring him to the surgery for X-ray a year later. The wing had healed well.

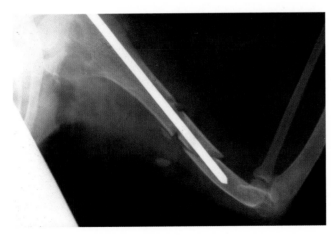

Surgery is nearly complete. The three pieces of bone have been restored to their natural position and held by a steel pin.

were still at the table in relaxed conversation. Then the telephone rang. I was on duty so I took the call.

"Hello, Neville, don't panic. I don't need a visit, just a bit of advice."

The voice was that of Adam, one of the many clients with whom I shared a good friendship.

"It's my drake," he said.

The problem was that Adam's best drake, "Daffy", had had an altercation with a Dales Pony, and, of course, had come off worst. Daffy's wing was obviously broken. My advice was being sought as to how the wing could be strapped or splinted.

Throughout my career I retained flushes of youthful optimism and enthusiasm, and I felt another one coming on. Here was an opportunity to tackle something I'd never done before: orthopaedic surgery on a duck! Adam was concerned about fees, but I assured him that this one was "on the house".

Half an hour later the patient arrived, and Robert and I were soon able to diagnose a serious fracture of the humerus, the long bone between the shoulder and elbow. Anaesthesia was going to be a problem, but we succeeded using an injectable drug normally used in cats. Daffy was soon relaxed, and the X-ray picture confirmed that two breaks had left the bone in three distinct pieces. It was shattered.

Daffy was sleeping soundly. While I prepared the instruments, Robert unceremoniously plucked the ailing wing, creating an unseasonal snowstorm of duck down in the prep room. This gave us a fit of the giggles before we settled down to the serious business of surgery.

Between us we dredged from our memories all we had learned in early days at college when "The Anatomy of the Fowl" had been studied. We cut successfully into the wing, circumventing several important-looking nerves and blood vessels, to expose the three distinct pieces of bone.

Having carefully measured the internal diameter of the bone, we chose a suitable stainless steel pin. These are rather like sturdy knitting needles, but with a sharp point on each end. The broken end of the top piece of bone, the one nearest the shoulder, was grasped, and the pin introduced into the marrow cavity. (Birds don't actually have a "marrow cavity" but it's best described that way.) The pin was driven carefully up towards the shoulder and out through the skin. By drawing most of the pin's length through the shoulder we could line up the other two pieces of bone, and push the pin down, impaling them in a straight line. With the bottom end of the pin firmly embedded in the dense bone near the elbow joint, we trimmed the pin and closed the wound.

Anaesthesia had been just right. Daffy gave a couple of sleepy disapproving quacks as we tied the last suture.

Elated by a highly successful piece of surgery, Robert and I drove home at about midnight. We chuckled at the thought of ridiculous consequences

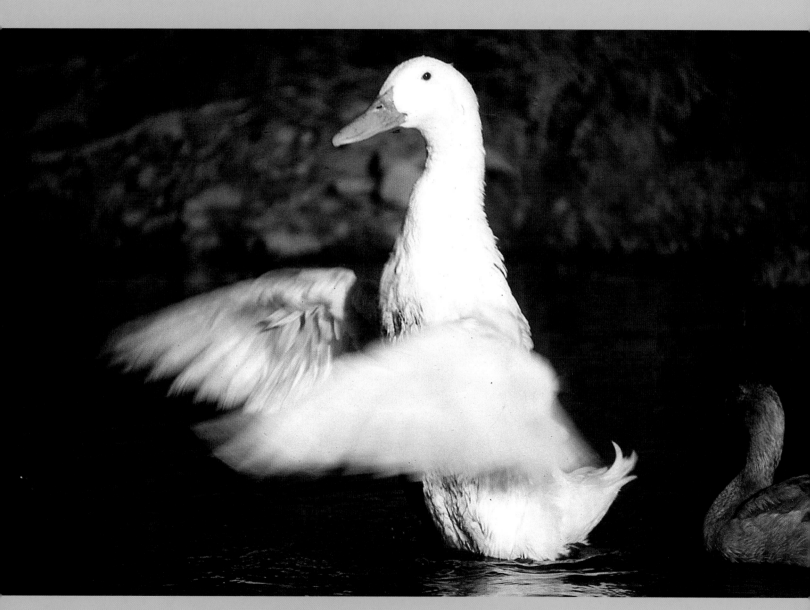

As if to announce that he was fully recovered, Daffy rose on the water and demonstrated two perfect wings.

of a duck with a lump of steel in one wing, and imagined poor old Daffy doing Eskimo rolls on the duck pond, or flying in ever-decreasing circles.

In fact, Daffy made a perfect recovery. A few weeks later, on a call to Adam's farm, we went down to the duck pond. As if to say "thank you", Daffy rose on the water and demonstrated two perfect wings.

There's a post-script to this tale. Just a few months later, a peregrine falcon was brought to the surgery.

It had been shot, and the humerus was in an even worse state than Daffy's. With experience of avian orthopaedics behind us, we performed another minor miracle. And that bird recovered fully and flew once more.

What fun it is being a vet!

19 Counting My Chickens

I really could not hazard a guess at the number of farmyards I have visited, but each has an ambience of its own. My favourites by far are those with a rich assortment of chickens, ducks, and geese adding their colour and character to the farmyard scene.

The poultry are traditionally fed and watered by the farmer's wife. They are her preserve, and in many cases, the nursery book picture of her scattering largesse to the ever-hungry birds is, in many cases, accurate.

It is generally accepted that chickens were first domesticated about five thousand years ago in India. There is evidence that they were in Egypt by 1400 BC, and arrived in Britain about two thousand years ago. All were developed from the Red jungle fowl. I find it fascinating that if left to breed randomly, the plumage of the offspring will, within just a few generations, tend to revert to the primaeval colours of its ancestor.

It is strange that from the earliest days of domestication through to Roman times, the breeding of fighting cocks was one of the most important aspects of poultry-keeping. Although the barbarism of cockfighting is now a thing of the past, magnificent specimens of "old English game" can be seen in many dales farmyards.

Cockfighting goes on in the farmyard all the time, but this is cockfighting as nature intended. It's all bluster. It ensures that the biggest and most vigorous

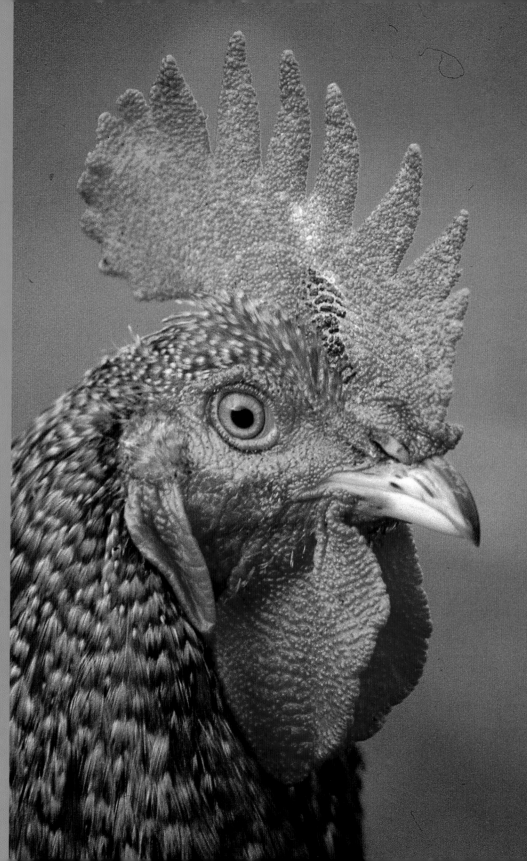

I loved farmyards with a colourful display of poultry. This picture was taken seconds after I'd stopped my car. I wound down the window, picked up my camera, and grabbed the shot.

cock birds are the winners, and the loser can slink away before any serious damage is done. Only the best specimens will have the opportunity to sire the next generation. It's sad that the barbarism of man once manipulated this instinctive behaviour by putting cocks specially bred for aggression into an arena from which there was no escape.

Many dales farmers were keen poultry enthusiasts. Having achieved success locally, it was common for these farmers and smallholders to exhibit nationally. How, I wondered, could this be achieved so long ago? The answer is obvious when one considers that in those days every small village had a railway station.

The railway companies operated a cheap and very efficient system whereby birds in their exhibition cages could be left at the station on the Friday afternoon and delivered to the Saturday show. At the show they were exhibited, fed, and watered, and returned to their proud owners on the Sunday. Even though this practice is obsolete, it is amusing to note that many current show catalogues still bear the legend, "Sorry, no rail traffic accepted."

I recently had the privilege of handling the old scrapbook of Wilf Parkin, a noted poultry enthusiast. It was from the era of "rail traffic", and

I was amazed to see prizewinning tickets from Oxford, Newark, Matlock, Liverpool, Bakewell, King's Lynn, Crystal Palace, and the National Dairy Show at Olympia.

Sadly, intensive poultry production in the second half of the twentieth century resulted in the decline of many of the once-famous breeds. The modern supermarket chicken or egg bears little resemblance to its handsome predecessors. Fortunately a handful of enthusiasts still keep the historic commercial breeds alive, and it is good to see that these handsome specimens are still well represented at the dales agricultural shows. The effort required to breed and show these birds is considerable, and it is all accomplished by enthusiasm.

I know all the farmyards that sport a colourful collection of poultry, and as I approach along the farm lane, I'm hoping to see a handsome cock bird posing on a wall or on the top spar of a gate. With camera at the ready and car window down, it's great fun trying to catch a spectacular pose. It's even more fun trying to capture the moment when he takes a deep breath and launches into a full-blown "cock-a-doodle-doo". My library has many an image that could grace the front of a packet of a well-known brand of cornflakes.

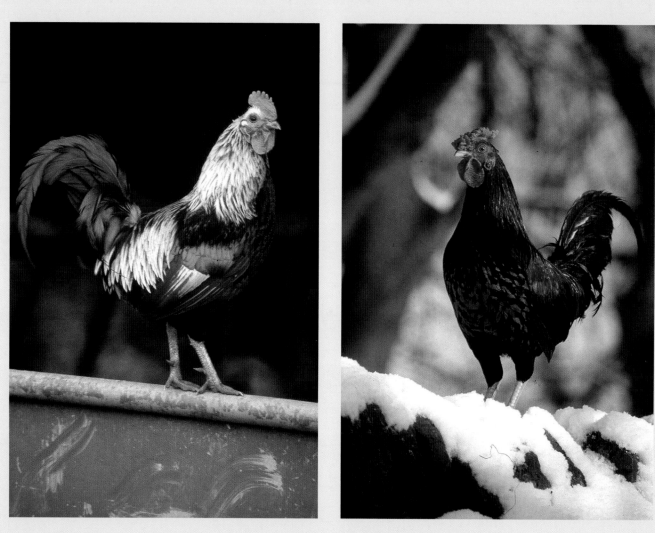

Approaching a farm, I was always on the lookout for a handsome cock bird perching on a gate or a wall.

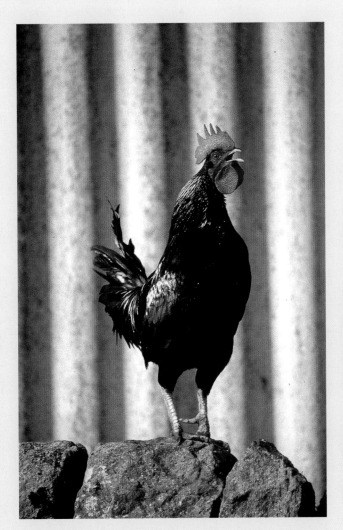
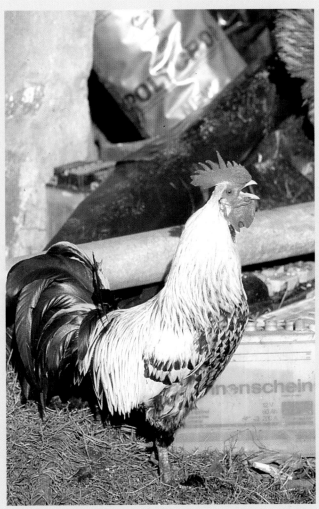

Having amassed a library of chicken portraits, the next challenge was to catch my subject in full-blown "cock-a-doodle-doo".

In today's modern high-tech farmyard, isn't it refreshing to find that caring attitudes prevail? The farmyard with poultry is one where colour and character are appreciated; where traditional values prosper; and where the farmer derives real pleasure from husbanding his stock.

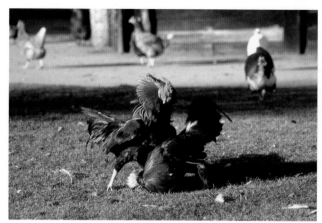

Cockfighting in the farmyard is colourful and dramatic, but it's all bluster. The loser will quit the engagement before any harm is done. Nature designed it that way. The biggest, most dominant bird will be the one who will pass on his genes . . .

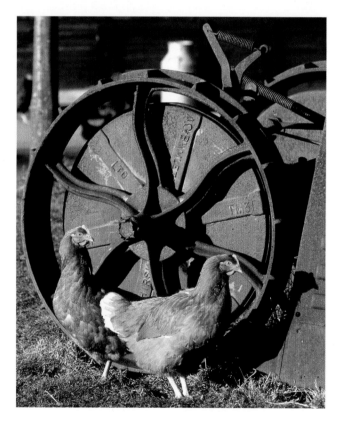

A typical farmyard scene with chickens.

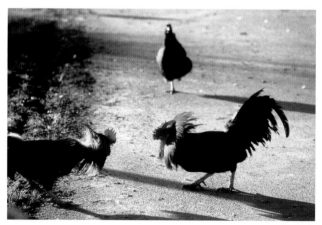

. . . and it's all because of a woman. She's lurking in the background!

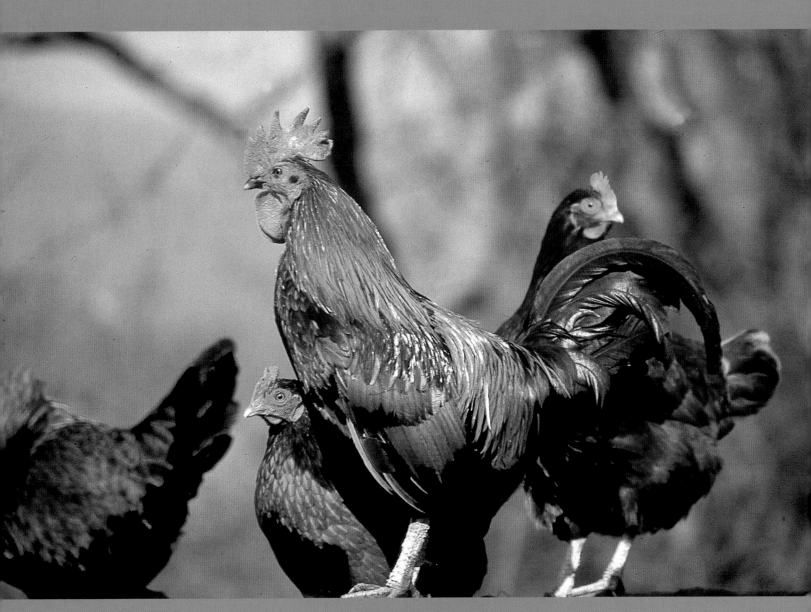

This cock bird demonstrates plumage that approximates to that of the Red jungle fowl, from which all modern poultry are descended.

20 The Duck with the Elvis Presley Hairstyle

I love living in Barnard Castle. It's a compact little dales market town, so virtually everyone lives within walking distance of the town centre.

One Saturday morning I was walking into town to do a bit of weekend shopping, and as I passed by the auction mart I noticed that it was a hive of activity. The car park was full to overflowing, and its environs were packed with people. Tuesdays and Wednesdays were the normal days for livestock sales and occasionally there would be a weekend sale of antiques or horticulture, but nowhere had I seen any publicity for this Saturday event.

It turned out to be a sale of "Rare and Minority Breed Poultry, Waterfowl, Poultry Equipment, and Cage Birds". During my years in practice I'd always loved the farmyards with the added colour of chickens, ducks, and geese, and so I decided to stay a while. I was intrigued by this huge assembly of enthusiasts.

Successful bidders scurried across the car park with their purchases. One, carrying a cage containing four guinea fowl, was highly delighted with his acquisition, and related excitedly his hopes that the warning calls of the birds would alert him to the presence of foxes in his farmyard.

The sale catalogue was a delight. Eighty-three vendors had come from as far afield as Dumfries, Wigton, Lancaster, Huddersfield, and Whitby, to present over three hundred lots.

As well as budgerigars, canaries, pigeons, quail, peafowl, and partridge, there were almost 600 chickens, 148 ducks, 28 geese, and 23 guinea fowl, a total of over 800 birds.

A bewildering assortment of breeds of chickens was on display, including such exotics as Salmon Favorolle, and Transylvanian Naked Necks. Duck breeds, too, were in abundance, with Muscovy, Aylesbury, Indian Runner, White Crested, Call Duck, Swedish Blue, Silver Appleyard, and Cayuga.

My particular favourite has got to be the Muscovy—a regular in the dales farmyards. Its size and bearing are so dramatic, and with a striking red face-mask and a hairstyle reminiscent of the Elvis Presley era it looks so very different from any other waterfowl.

It therefore comes as no surprise to find that the Muscovy is, literally, a breed apart with a distinct genetic make-up. It is the only domesticated duck with no wild mallard blood in its ancestry. Crossing Muscovies with mallard types is possible, but they

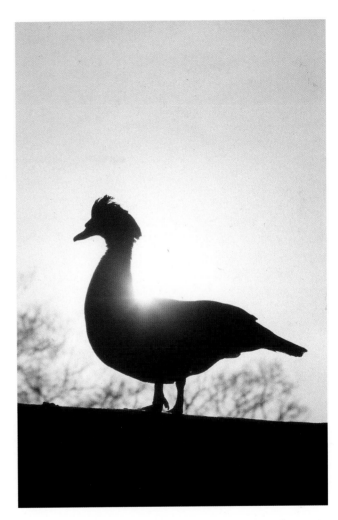

A silhouette at sunset. There's no mistaking the subject.

The Duck with the Elvis Presley Hairstyle   137

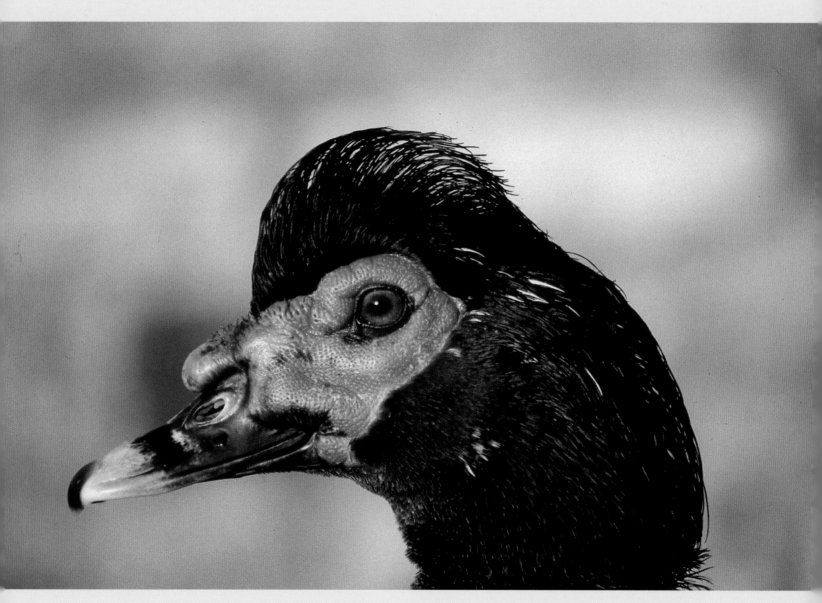

The flamboyant bird with the flamboyant hairstyle.

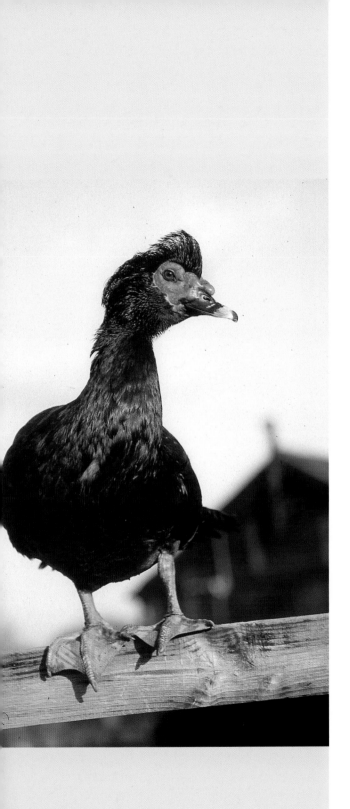

are so genetically distinct that the offspring are always sterile.

The Muscovy female is a wonderful mother. I remember arriving at a farm and noticing a bizarre sight. In an orchard, under an apple tree a Muscovy mum was incubating her eggs in a wooden tomato box. The farmer explained that he had been clearing overgrown ivy from the garden wall and in doing so had inadvertently disturbed the duck, which was sitting on eggs. Eggs and downy nest lining were scattered far and wide. All he could do to save the situation was to gather up the down and the eggs, and arrange them in an old tomato box that happened to be lying close by.

Within minutes the duck had waddled over to the box, inspected the eggs, and resumed her incubating duties as though nothing had happened.

The maternal devotion continues after the eggs have hatched. The ducklings follow her everywhere, not only staying in close contact, but communicating with soft cheeps and quacks. Should danger threaten, mother will hiss aggressively and fluff up her plumage to make herself look large and fearsome. At the same time she manages to shepherd her little flock away from the threat and into cover.

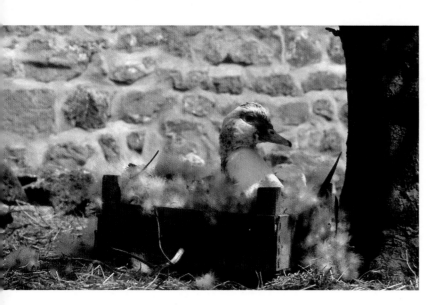

Having accidentally destroyed the nest, the farmer reconstructed it in a tomato box and replaced the eggs. It says much for the mothering instinct of the Muscovy, that she inspected the new "nest" and eggs, then continued incubating them as though nothing had happened.

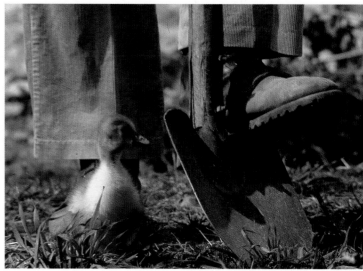

The phenomenon of imprinting. This little Muscovy adopted the farmer's boots as its mother.

Like most waterfowl, there is a strong imprinting instinct in the Muscovy. Imprinting is the mechanism where, at the point of hatching, the first moving thing the duckling sees becomes its image of the mother figure. It will follow that figure doggedly wherever it goes and it is this imprinting that gave rise to another amusing encounter with a Muscovy.

Arriving at a farm, I was again confronted by a bizarre sight. The farmer was digging his vegetable garden, and running in and out between the spade and the farmer's boots was a Muscovy duckling.

This little fellow had emerged from the egg long after Mum had collected her newly hatched ducklings together and left the nest site with her brood. The first moving object that the duckling saw was the farmer's boots walking past, and they had become the object of its imprinting instinct.

Everywhere the boots went, the duckling followed. When the farmer returned to the farmhouse and took off his boots by the back door, the duckling just snuggled down beside them. As amusing as the tale is, it had a sad end, for, as you can imagine, the orphan duck with a boot as a parent turned out to be a very mixed-up Muscovy.

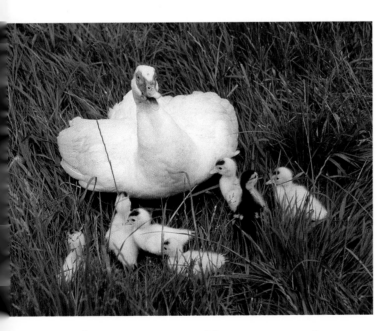

Mother Muscovy sees me with my camera as a threat to her family so she puffs herself up and hisses angrily.

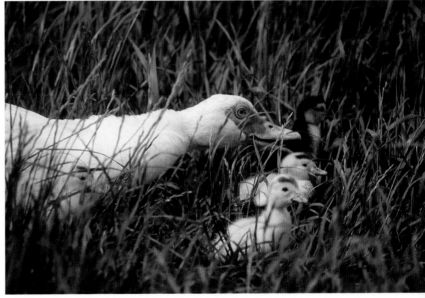

When the intruder refuses to go away, she shepherds her precious ducklings to safety in the long grass.

21 Why did the Owl 'Owl?

S o ran a conundrum in a Christmas cracker that I pulled several years ago.

In that context it's a bit of a silly question, but in reality it's not all that silly.

Owls, worldwide, are a vociferous race, and you don't have to live in the countryside to be familiar with the nocturnal hooting and screeching of your local tawny owl population. The tawny owl is as much at home in urban parkland and wooded suburbs as it is in the open countryside.

Here is a sensible answer to the apparently silly question in the title. The owl noises you hear are part of a rich vocabulary which maintains the social structure in your area. They use it to delineate

territories and establish pair bonds in the prelude to the breeding season. Fledglings and adults maintain animated "conversation" throughout the hours of darkness.

When you hear an owl hoot, you may hear answering calls from several other individuals at varying distances and directions from the originator of the conversation. The female makes the "Tu-whit", while the male responds with a low hoot (commonly described as "Tu-whoooo"). There are lots more noises in the vocabulary, some executed in flight.

Caring for wildlife casualties was an exciting and very rewarding part of my professional life. I even built an aviary in my back garden for accommodation

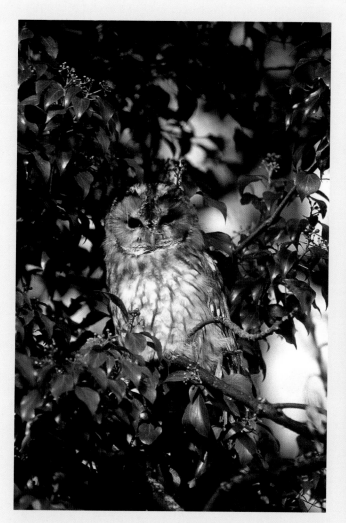

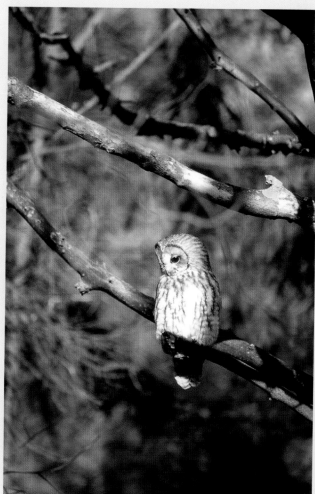

Tawny owls are birds of the woodland.

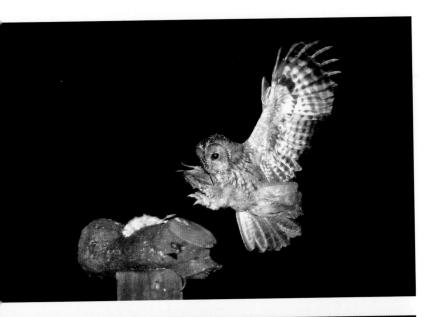

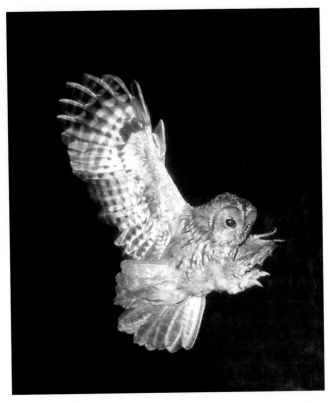

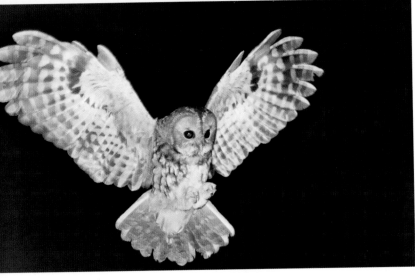

This bird visits our garden every evening. We suspect that it's one that we cared for and released many years ago. Occasionally we provide him with a snack.

and rehabilitation. I must have attended hundreds of wildlife cases, but without doubt, the tawny owl dominated the caseload. Abandoned fledglings, broken wings, and concussion from collision with motor cars were the main problems.

My colleagues and I learned a little more from every case that came through our hands, and although we would never claim to be experts, our success rate has been high.

On one occasion we had three tawnies in the aviary and another one was brought to the surgery. His concussion was slight, and we knew he just needed twenty-four hour's rest and a good feed. But how would we identify him next day? Chris had a great idea. She painted a few of his talons with nail varnish before we put him in the aviary. This enabled us to catch him next day and release him with the minimum of fuss. How we chuckled at the thought of a tawny owl flying through the woods, sporting talons in a delicate shade of pink.

Over the years we have reared and released lots of fledglings. Baby owls leave the nest when quite young, probably little more than three weeks old, but they are watched over and fed by diligent parents for several more weeks. Whenever a baby owl was brought to us we would try to ascertain where it was found. After checking it over we would return it to its home patch, placing it on a low branch away from predators. There its parents would be sure to locate it and resume their duties.

The youngsters have a particularly plaintive "I'm hungry" call, which the parents cannot ignore.

Where relocation was not possible, we would assume responsibility for overseeing the transformation of a little ball of fluff into a handsome adult bird. At this stage it is very easy to convince the baby that you are its mum and dad. This "imprinting" must be avoided at all costs if the owl is to lead a normal life in the wild. Imprinted birds, on release, can pester and attack people for the rest of their lives.

Once we almost had an imprinting incident. One of our releases used to come back now and again to say "Hi". He would fly into the garden, sometimes perching on the bird table, and chatter to us. He was obviously hunting and feeding well since he was in fine condition. We never fed him, and his visits became less and less frequent as he matured.

Another of our little orphans was extremely fortunate.

Shortly after he moved into the aviary he was adopted by a pair of tawny owls who were rearing their young in the woods at the bottom of our garden. Although he was not one of theirs, the plaintive "I'm hungry" calls and their parental instincts had convinced them otherwise. Even in

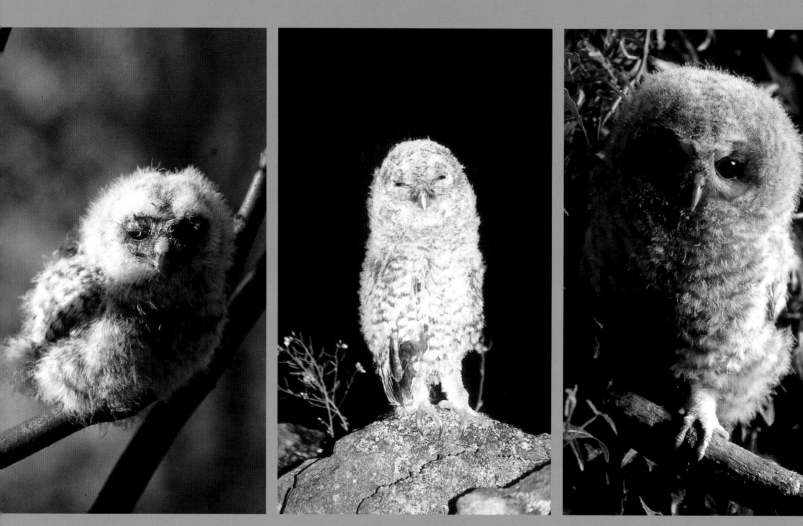

Tawny owl chicks may not be very pretty, but . . .

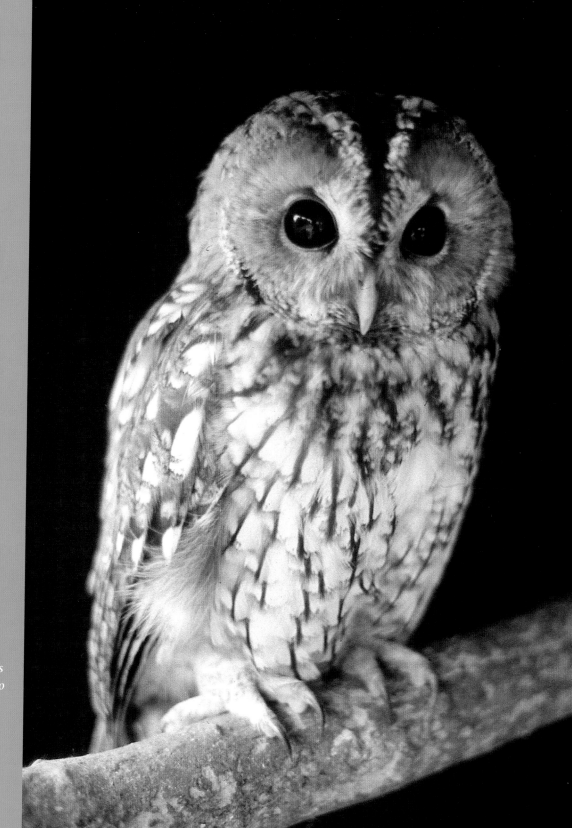

. . . like Hans Christian Andersen's ugly duckling, each will grow up to be a beautiful "swan".

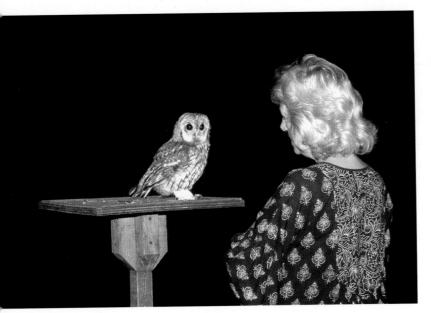

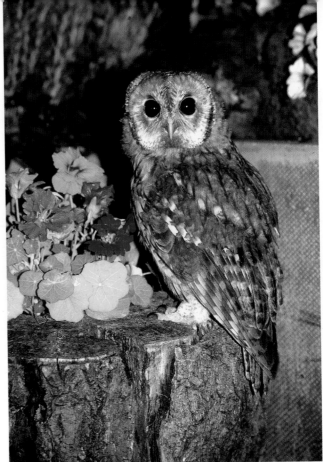

This owl, after we had reared it and released it, would call to see us occasionally. Although it was tempting to encourage the friendship, we didn't feed him. He had obviously learned to hunt, as he was in perfect condition. His visits became less and less frequent as he resumed life in the wild.

daylight hours they would fly in with their prey: rats, mice, frogs, and small birds.

The prey would be passed through the weldmesh to the hungry youngster. If it was too big to pass through, they would perch on the roof of the aviary and reduce it to smaller portions then pass the pieces through, one by one. As soon as he developed flight feathers, we released him in the woods to join his foster parents and brothers and sisters.

And one final tale.

Several years ago, in the depths of winter, we saw a tawny owl perching high in an ash tree at the bottom of the garden. As we looked at him, he calmly returned our stare. I mentioned to Chris that perhaps he had been one of our patients.

Chris suggested that I should put a chick (we keep a supply of day-old chicks in the freezer for our patients) on the bird table. If he was one of ours, he would probably come down and take it.

And so I did. And within seconds he swooped down to collect his free supper. Since then he calls regularly. We don't always feed him, but we do from time to time, especially in the spring when he has a hungry family to feed. As he gained in confidence, he would take off from his high perch with immaculate timing and silent wings, to pick up the chick as soon as I had placed it. It was an amazing feeling, being within three feet of a wild tawny owl and feeling the draught from his wings as he turned for the woods, clutching his supper.

I could go on. There are so many stories to tell.

But in case you'd like to hear the answer to "Why did the owl 'owl?". . .

It's because the woodpecker would peck 'er.

Get it?

22 The Starling's Amazing Story

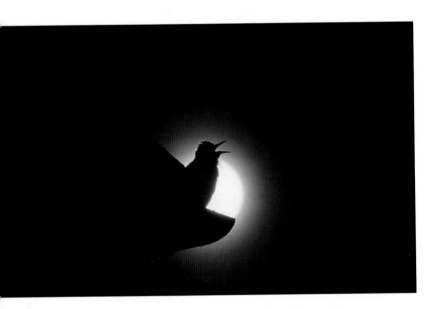

A starling sits on the corner of our house. His merry chuckling and warbling announces that this is his patch and he's setting up home here.

Many years ago, whilst on holiday on Holy Island, a very excited young man spotted the binoculars around my neck and assumed that I was a fellow "twitcher".

"Have you seen the barred warbler?" he enquired. His high excitement was in no way dented by my negative reply.

"Well, have you seen the glaucous gull?" he continued. Another negative reply failed to dampen his enthusiasm.

"What about the red-backed shrike?" was his final attempt to share with me his enjoyment of a successful day's bird-watching.

I tell this story to illustrate the diversity of enjoyment that can be gained from an interest in the natural world. I genuinely admired the young man's knowledge and dedication, but I get my kicks watching and learning about the more familiar species.

Every working day I was able to observe starlings. Most farmsteads had a resident colony. Wherever I travelled there were always starlings somewhere in view, and I was able to make a special study of their movements and behavioural patterns.

Man has played a huge part in the success of the species. Five thousand years ago, when Neolithic man came to a densely forested northern Europe, he started chopping down trees, removing countless nesting sites. But in doing so, he created millions of acres of short-cropped grassland, the ideal feeding grounds for the birds. At the same time he began building houses, with eaves and nooks and crannies, which replaced the primaeval nest sites. The bird still lives in close proximity to man.

I find every aspect of the bird's lifestyle fascinating.

For instance, next time you see starlings feeding on your lawn, take a closer look. Their pecking is a very specialised form of food gathering, made

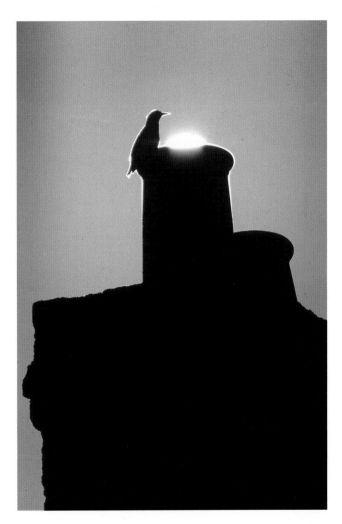

Since Stone Age man cleared the forest to provide vast areas of short-cropped grassland, and built houses with nooks and crannies to provide nest sites, the starling has lived in close proximity to man.

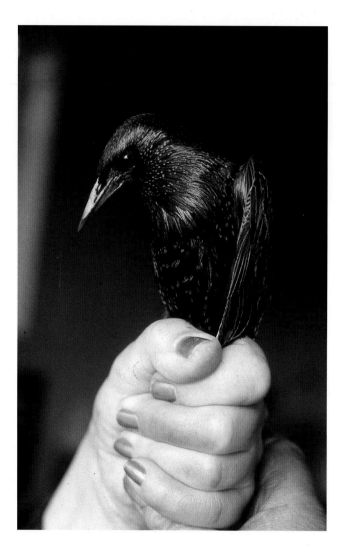

possible by ingenious design of the skull. It's a brilliant example of nature's engineering. The strong beak is plunged into the sward. Powerful muscles then open the beak. At the same time the eyes rotate forwards and outwards to see what food has been exposed. During the summer months this feeding method turns up a plentiful supply of leatherjackets, the larvae of crane flies, (daddy-long-legs). During winter months the starling adapts its diet to include fruits, berries, and seeds.

I had often come across an intact starling egg on the hard surfaces of roads, footpaths, and in farmyards. I once saw such a discarded egg impaled on a metal gate. The egg had obviously been deposited intact on the roof of the barn and had rolled off, to land on the gate.

It puzzled me as to how this came about and I discovered that the answer lies in a strange behaviour pattern in the laying female. Occasionally she will visit a neighbouring nest and remove an egg, placing it carefully at a distance before returning to lay one of her eggs in the neighbour's nest.

After twelve days' incubation the eggs hatch. The chick is a mere fifth of an ounce, and is totally naked and helpless. Twelve days later the chick

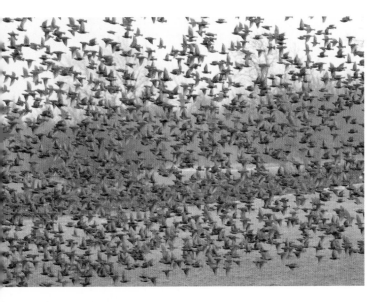

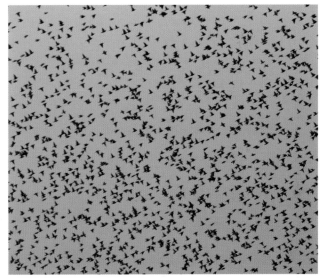

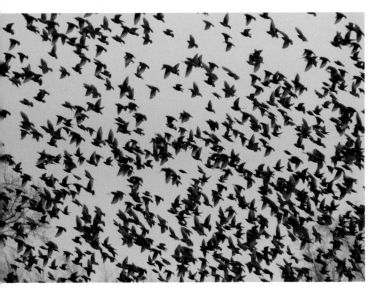

Watching a flock of starlings lift off from the pastures en masse is an amazing sight. It's done in perfect synchrony. Soon the sky is full of starlings.

has increased its bodyweight twelve times to two and a half ounces, and is fully feathered. That's a staggering growth rate fuelled by a constant supply of high-protein, high-water-content leatherjackets.

The young leave the nest at twenty-one days. For a week or so the demanding adolescents continue to be fed by parents before embarking on a precarious state of independence. In a very short time they must become streetwise. Sixty to seventy per cent

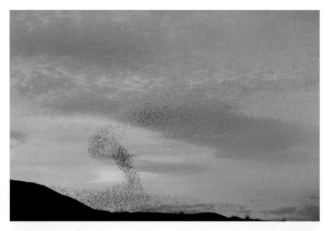

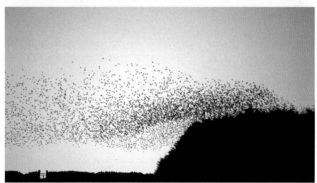

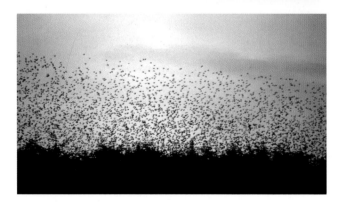

As the murmuration approaches the roost site, it wheels around the sky before pouring itself into the treetops.

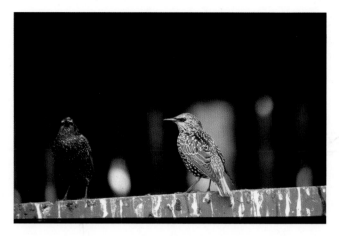

Starlings moult once a year, in October, into this spotty plumage. There is no further moult. The glossy summer plumage appears as the white tips on the feathers wear away.

of these young birds will perish in their first year. This naivety was vividly illustrated one summer's evening when I arrived at a farmyard, and was accosted by a fledgling starling. In the absence of his parents he rushed up to me, demanding food. It was a great photo opportunity, but made difficult by his trotting towards me and perching on my lens! Each time I gently cast him away he would look more and more perplexed, before galloping back to perch on my lens again. Eventually he got the message, but if it had been the farmyard cat he had accosted instead of me, he would have become a mortality statistic.

As late summer progresses into autumn, the social nature of the starling can be seen in the spectacular congregations in night roosts. Several years ago a

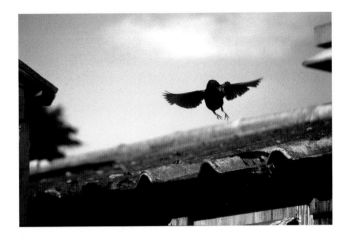

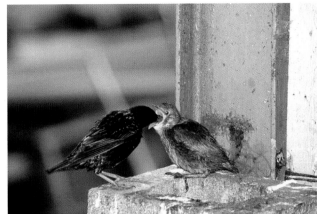

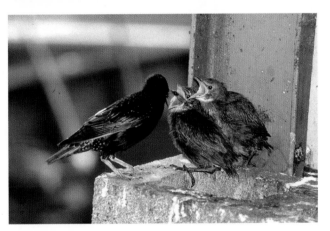

Feeding the young is a full-time job from dawn till dusk. Leatherjackets (daddy-long-legs larvae) are an important food source providing fluid and protein to fuel the rapid growth rate of the chicks.

night roost established itself in a conifer plantation at the top of the dale. Fascinated by this daily forty-mile round trip, I followed a day-feeding flock on its twenty-mile journey from my home town to the roost site. Throughout the journey the flock was joined by other groups, so that by the time it had reached the conifer plantation, numbers had increased from a few hundred individuals to several thousand, and they finally alighted on pastures near the night roost. There they took a bite of supper while further clouds of birds appeared from all points of the compass till the pastures were black with starlings taking a final feed before turning in.

And then, as though a secret signal had been given, the fields were green again. It was now the sky that was darkened by thousands of birds wheeling and undulating en masse before pouring themselves into the dark treetops. The amazing in-flight co-ordination of the immense "murmuration" is one of the wonders of nature. Scientists have recently discovered how they do it. It appears that each bird takes a "fix" on the seven individuals nearest to it. Thus there is an interlocking mass of units of seven birds, which gives thousands of birds the appearance of acting as a single organism.

The reasons for this daily forty-mile round trip are obscure. Nature seldom runs up an expenditure of energy without advantages. It's likely that the answer is complicated. Most natural phenomena defy a simple one-word explanation.

And a final thought.

The starling population has been in steep decline in recent years. I have noticed that at the same time, the annual autumn invasion of our house by "daddy-long-legs" has declined too. If there's

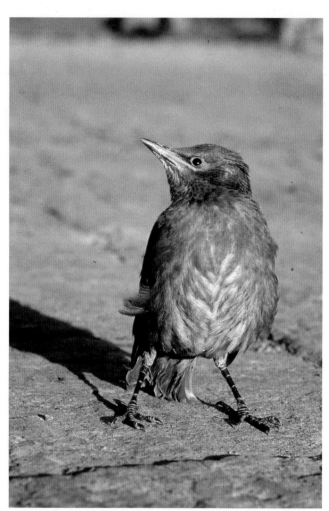

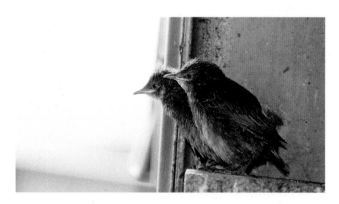

These two ingénues are at the point of fledging. Within a day or two they will have to learn to look after themselves. Sadly, many will perish.

I met this little chap in a farmyard one evening. He came running up to me, thinking I might feed him. If I had been the farmyard cat, he would have been in big trouble. I do hope he soon learned to be a little more streetwise.

a shortage of daddy-long-legs, there will be a shortage of leatherjackets, which are the starling's staple summer food as well as being essential for rearing a healthy brood. Could it be that the two are connected in another of nature's multifactorial mysteries?

I call this my Icarus picture because these starlings seem to be flying into the sun. According to Greek mythology, Daedalus and his son Icarus built wings with wax and feathers to escape from Crete. In spite of his father's warnings, Icarus flew too near to the sun, the wax melted, and he perished.

23 The Year of the Grouse

Virtually every working day my journeys took me across the heather moors of the high Pennines. In the spring thousands of songbirds and waders flock to these hills to breed. It is so exciting to watch the sights and sounds of their frantic summer activity. Their stay seems so brief, because once their parental duties are over, it appears they waste no time in leaving the moor.

And so, between September and February the heather moors are almost totally abandoned. Only the red grouse remains. He is welded to these moors and will never leave unless conditions become desperate. It is perhaps because of the resilience of the bird and the fact that it's always there that I have developed a special interest in its natural history, and since the cock birds are vigorously territorial, it was possible to get to know the territories and habits of individual birds.

January and February can be the cruelest of months for the grouse on the high moors. Since their staple diet is heather shoots, substantial snowfall can separate the bird from its main food source. In January 1986, after a heavy fall of snow, there followed a succession of freezing and thawing. This resulted in the formation of a deep, impenetrable crust of ice over the whole moor. In places it was five inches thick.

Hundreds of birds stood about on the ice looking weak and bewildered. They were starving.

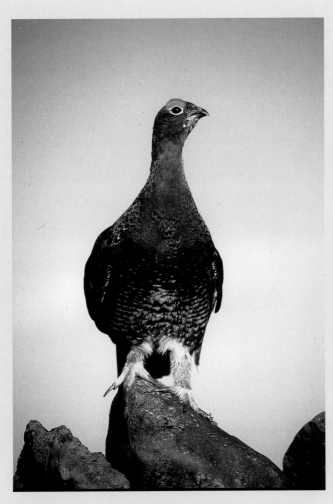

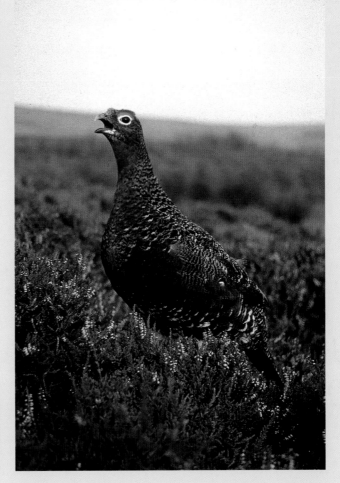

The cock bird in full dress uniform. Who could fail to be fascinated by such a handsome fellow?

In the summer he keeps a low profile, engaging in diligent family duties. After the moult in late summer there is a Jekyll and Hyde transformation. He wants the world to know he's there. From a high point in the middle of his chosen territory he watches for intruders.

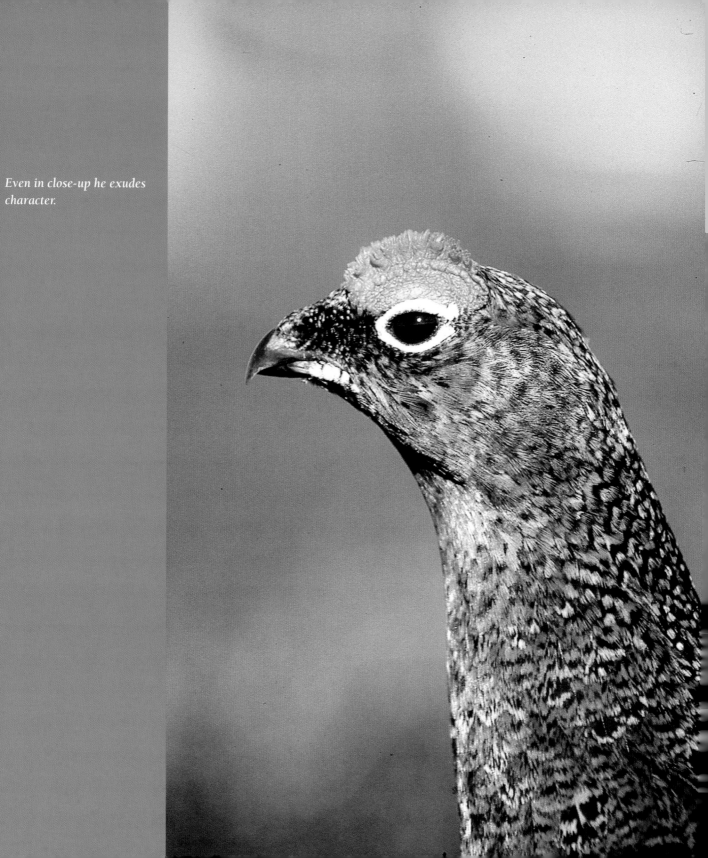

Even in close-up he exudes character.

Occasionally a huge flock would take to the air and wheel around the moor like a murmuration of starlings as they searched in vain for a break in the frozen surface.

Enterprising gamekeepers used all manner of mechanical aids to alleviate the situation. A local keeper drove for hours on a snow-sledge breaking the crust. Others used quad bikes, while some towed a harrow behind a tractor. The grouse were quick to take advantage of their efforts, and flocked in to the exposed heather like gulls behind a plough.

The spectacular territorial song-flight of the cock reaches a climax in March. A flight to the edge of the territory is followed by a vertical soar and a noisy descent as he confronts the tenant of the adjacent property. There follows a great deal of strutting and cussing at each other along the invisible boundary line before an equally flamboyant return to a prominent spot in the centre of their respective territories.

The hen has already moulted into camouflaged plumage. He now begins to moult into a duller and less obvious livery so that the pair can keep a low profile on the moor as they raise their family.

In May the chicks appear. From day one the precocious brown and olive mottled chicks fend for themselves. They are anxiously guarded and shepherded by both parents who instinctively take them to boggy areas of the moor where high-protein, easily digested insect food is available. Only gradually will the juvenile alimentary system adapt to the course fibrous diet of heather shoots. The parents are on constant watch for predators, and will fiercely attack creatures much larger than themselves to protect their brood.

I once watched a stoat approaching a family of poults but the hen bird was having none of it. She flew at the invader in a frenzy each time he tried to make an attack. He tried coming at the family from all angles, but eventually gave up.

A keeper once told me of a buzzard which flew too close to a grouse family. The hen bird took off and engaged the raptor in a spirited aerial dogfight, which, in spite of his huge size advantage, the buzzard lost.

The chicks grow apace. In the first week or two the hen will brood and protect the youngsters, then rise to allow a brief feeding foray. At a word from her, the recall will summon them back to the warmth and security of her body. A cold, wet May and June can be disastrous for these little fellows.

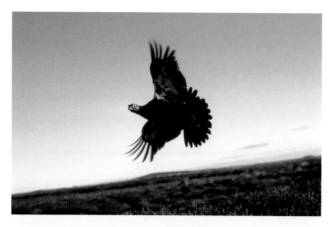

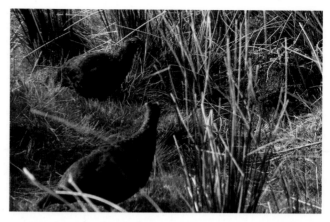

The noisy confrontation at the border of the territory.

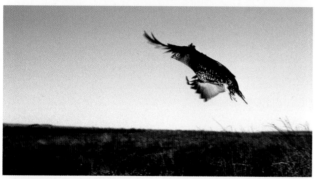

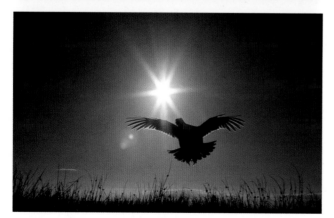

At the approach of an intruder he makes a noisy display flight to confront the interloper.

By the end of July the chicks reach adult weight and plumage. Over the next few months the small family groups tend to merge into larger packs. At the same time the cock bird's family instincts wane and give way to territorial existence. He moults into full dress uniform. The older, more dominant cocks will set up territories much larger than the average five acres. The younger cocks will have to make do with less. Some of the younger cocks who cannot establish territories are destined to perish over the winter.

Autumn territories and pair bonds will be maintained over the winter if the weather stays mild. Should the weather be severe, the cocks will abandon their chosen domains and join the packs. As soon as there is an improvement in conditions, they will be the first to leave the group.

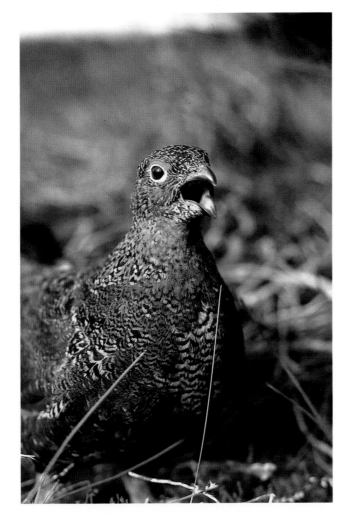

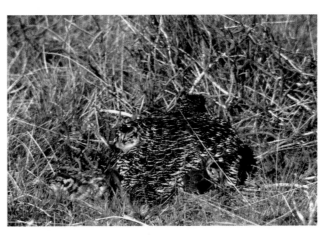

For the first week or so the hen will brood her chicks.

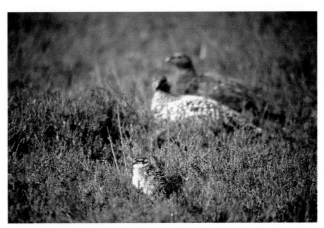

As they meet, there is open hostility. I'm sure they are using bad language!

Both parents diligently shepherd the chicks around the moor, on constant lookout for danger.

And so the cycle is complete. The proud and resilient species has triumphed over disease, predation, and climate. He'll be there to welcome his summer visitors next spring.

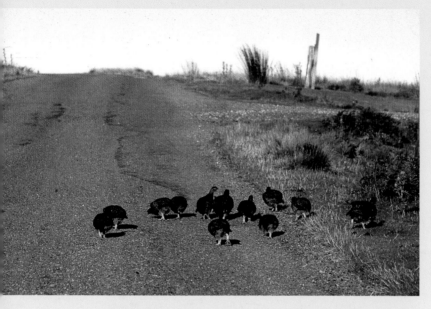

By the end of July the young are fully grown. There are ten poults and two adults in this picture, and it's hard to differentiate between them.

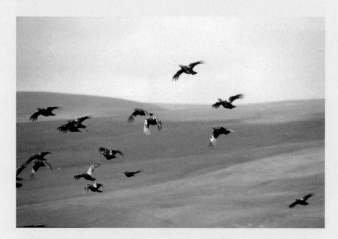

A pack of grouse fly across the moor.

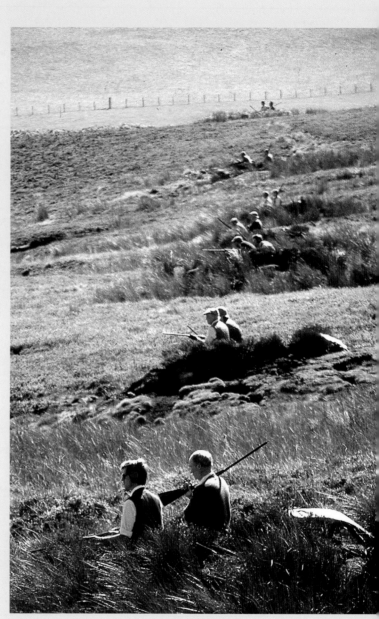

The shooting season.

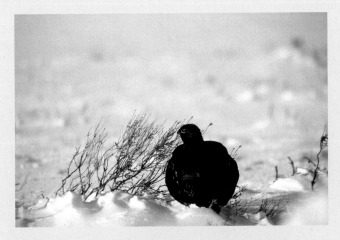

Harsh winters will separate the grouse from their food source. The exposed heather here has been stripped of all its shoots.

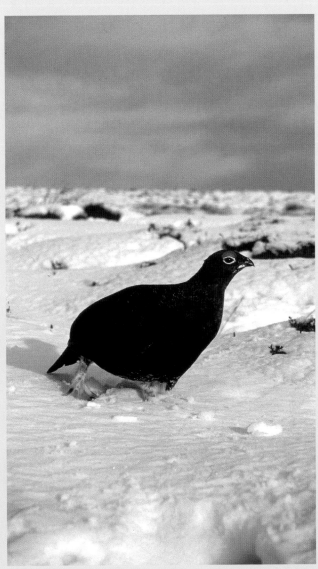

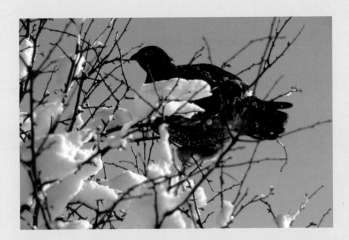

Although heather shoots are preferred, the grouse will make use of any available vegetation, including buds on the hawthorn trees at the edge of the moor.

At the end of a harsh spell of weather the cock is quick to break away from the winter congregations to re-establish his territory.

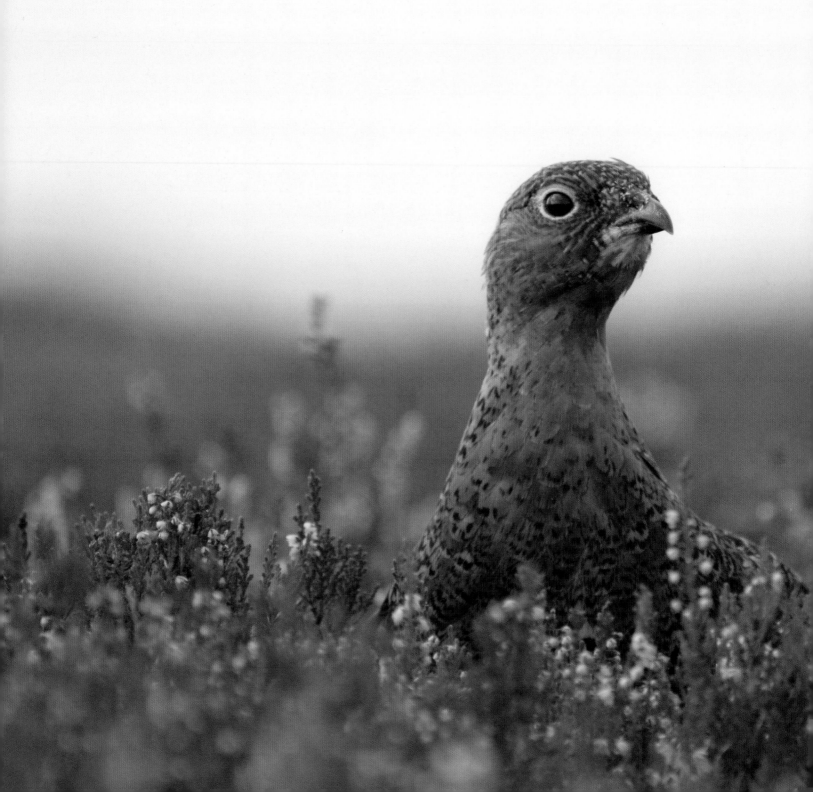

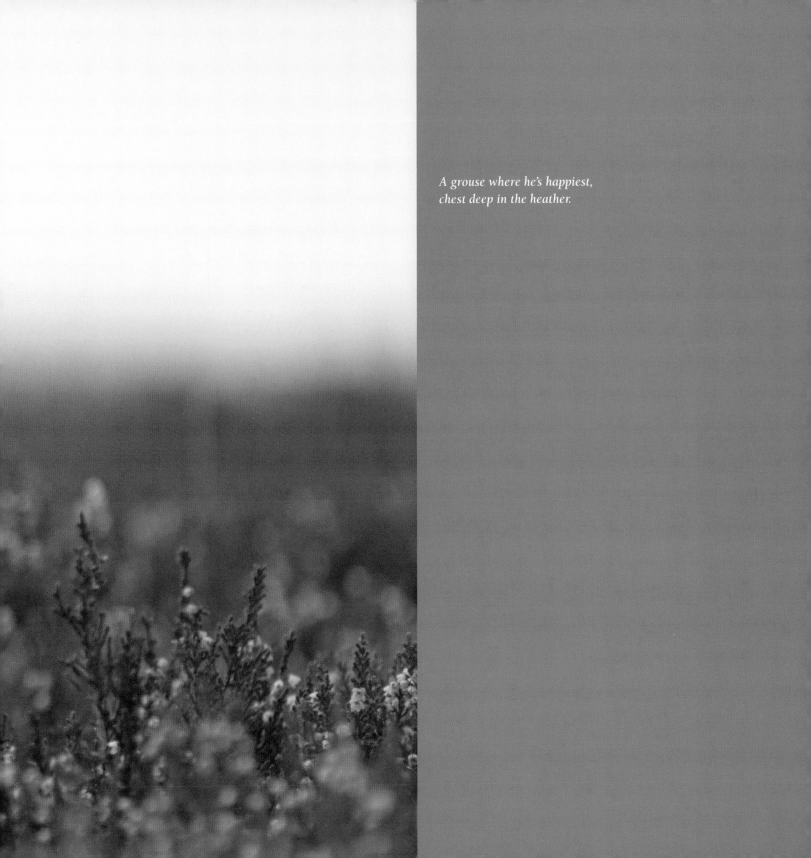

A grouse where he's happiest,
chest deep in the heather.

24 The Flying Squad

Many years ago I was driving around the dale on a working day and had a serious fit of the giggles. As usual, I was listening to Radio 2, and Terry Wogan, with his superb sense of the ridiculous, had suggested that a surefire winner in the TV ratings would be a vet cooking a meal while his house and garden were being given a makeover.

My imagination, and a sense of the ridiculous on a par with Wogan, could not help but picture the chaotic scenario. What he was really saying, of course, was that if you took away programmes about DIY, gardening, cooking, and vets, there would be a huge gap in the TV schedules. And it's still true today, thirty years on. Obviously I like to watch the veterinary programmes,

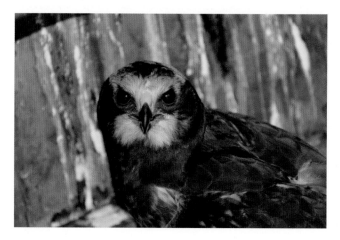

A marsh harrier which was brought to us with hardly any signs of life. She had so little flesh that she felt like a feather duster. She had been shot, and I had my doubts whether she would ever fly again. After months of care she was released on an RSPB reserve and immediately started quartering and hunting.

but my favourites by far are those that feature wildlife.

Every country practice has a steady stream of wildlife cases presented at reception. Most will, without hesitation, treat the injured creature at their own expense, and we were no exception. (Surely it would be boorish to send a bill to the Good Samaritan who had effected the rescue?)

Having had a great interest in natural history from childhood, I was positively excited at the prospect of handling and caring for these cases. In the early years we were "flying by the seat of our pants", but our knowledge was augmented by every patient's treatment and nursing techniques.

It was important to recognise the hopeless case and to identify where painless euthanasia was the only option. However, if I had a professional weakness, it was youthful optimism. Nothing beat the thrill of returning a physically sound patient to the wild after weeks, or perhaps months, of careful treatment.

Over the years I was privileged to count among my patients badgers, foxes, roe deer, all five species of British owl, hawks, falcons, buzzards, ducks, swans, woodpeckers, and even a mistle thrush.

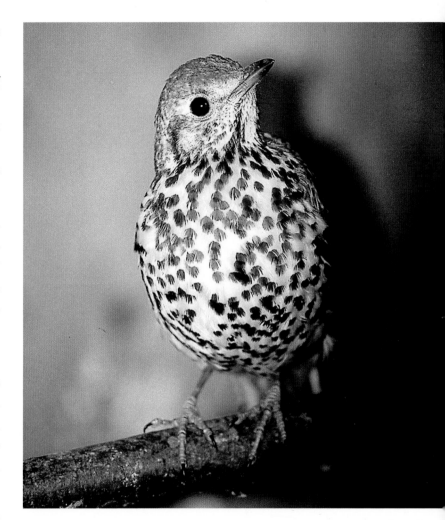

We reared this mistle thrush from fledgling through to adulthood, but he proved a costly patient. We had to line the aviary with chicken wire to stop him poking his head through the bars to say "hello" to our cats.

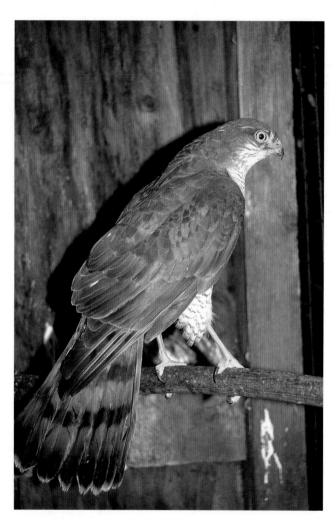

A sparrow hawk. These are difficult patients, refusing to feed and hurling themselves at the bars of the aviary. This one, however, got his act together and made a full recovery.

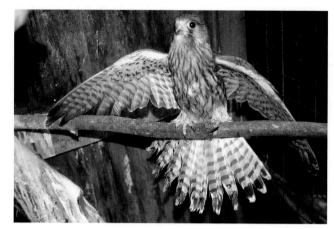

A kestrel.

The mistle thrush was brought to the surgery as an abandoned fledgling, not quite able to look after himself yet. He was happy in the aviary, and I dug over most of our garden to find food for him, but there was a problem. He behaved as everybody's friend. This included thrusting his head through the weldmesh of the aviary to say "Hi" to our two cats. The solution was to buy a roll of chicken wire (for £40!!) and line the aviary. Eventually he became quite mature and independent. It was a delight to release him in a part of the dale where there were lots of mistle thrushes, and he made a beeline to join a group of his own kind.

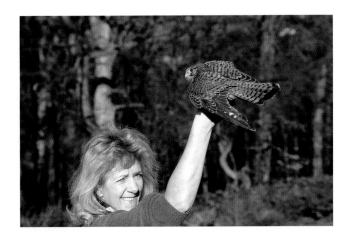

Chris releasing a kestrel.

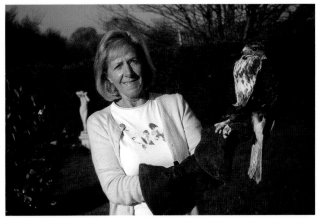

Chris releasing a buzzard.

Raptors are rather special. They are finely tuned flying machines and it is important to be sure that they are restored to a hundred per cent efficiency before releasing them. Anything less and their ability to hunt will be compromised, leading to a slow death by starvation. It is therefore a heavy responsibility deciding when to let them go.

My first major success was with a peregrine falcon. A peppering of shot from some vandal's twelve-bore had shattered its humerus, the long bone between shoulder and elbow. It took two hours of surgery to fix the bone, but a few weeks later it was flying again. What a delight. It's fortunate that no one had told me that two hours of anaesthesia is fatal in a bird of prey!

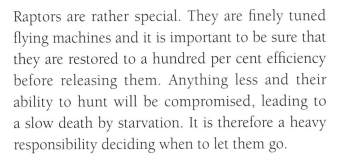

Chris releasing a sparrow hawk.

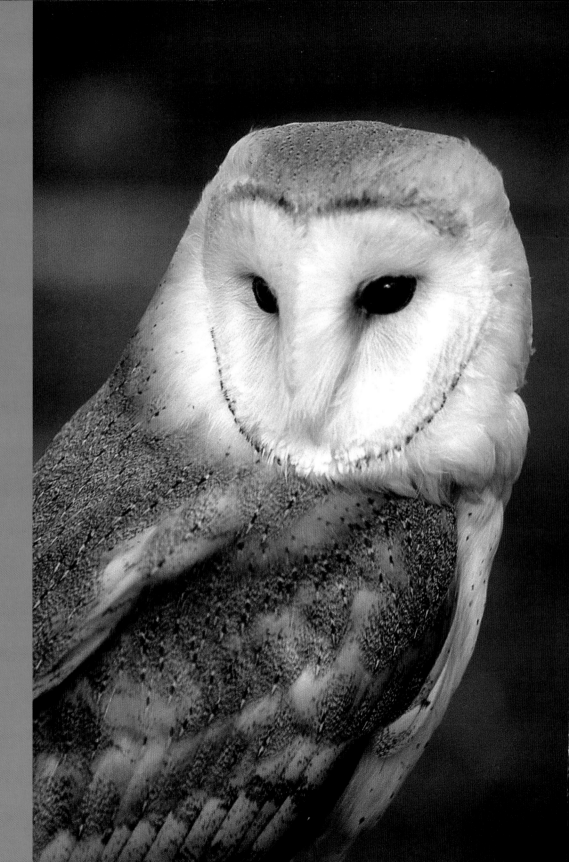

Barn owls are seen in increasing numbers in the dales after an almost complete absence.

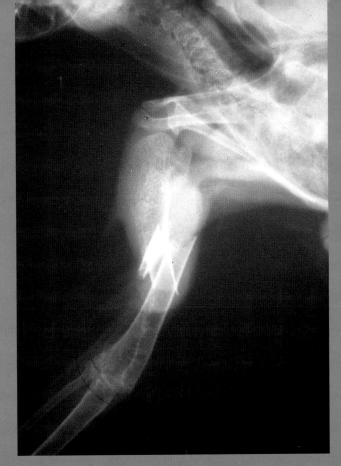

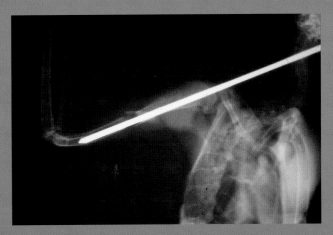

This is an X-ray of a barn owl who had a bad fracture of the humerus. (Very much like Daffy in my "Oh for the wings of a duck" story.) It was probably the result of a collision with a motor vehicle.

Surgery to pin the humerus.

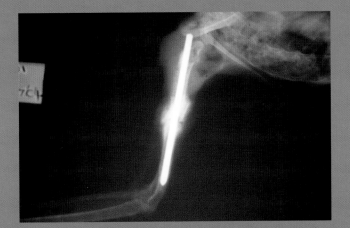

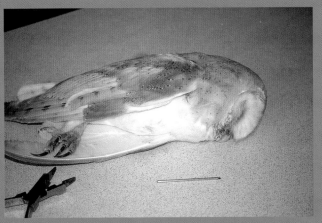

Less than three weeks later, an X-ray revealed complete healing so we removed the pin while the bird was still under anaesthetic.

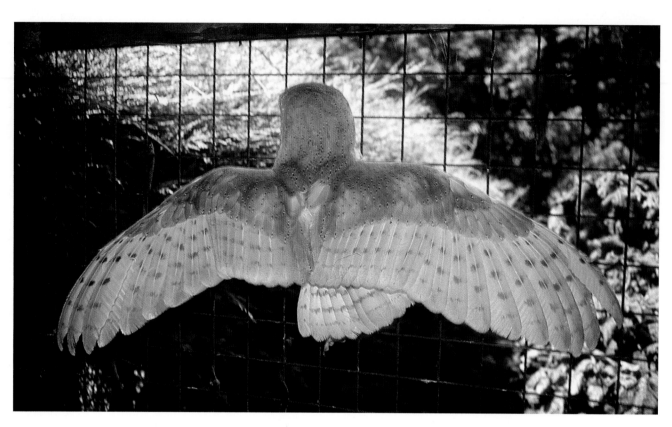

After a spell in the aviary he was flying well.

A marsh harrier was brought in to the surgery by a farmer's son. It was almost dead, showing no reaction. There was not an ounce of flesh on it. It was rather like handling a feather duster. Over a period of days careful rehydration and hand feeding restored its strength, and when it was fit enough we X-rayed it. It had been shot. The mid shaft of the humerus was reduced to powder, and although there was not much displacement, the soft tissue damage must have been enormous. I despaired of ever releasing this patient. However, because of the minimal displacement, and against the odds, nature healed the wing without any surgical interference. Months later it was released on a local RSPB reserve with extensive reedbeds. Within minutes it was hunting and quartering its favoured habitat.

The merlin is the smallest of European falcons, scarcely bigger than a blackbird. The Northern Pennines are a stronghold of this non-too-common species. A patient with a broken metacarpal (the tiny bone no wider than a piece of fuse wire which supports the flight feathers) was presented to us. After twenty-four hours of fluids and feeding we considered it a suitable case for surgery. I took charge of the anaesthesia while my colleague Paul (who's a "whizz" at orthopaedics) used a needle-fine stainless steel pin to stabilise the bone.

The patient was confined to a small cage to restrict movement and allow the wing to heal. Three weeks later the pin was removed: it looked good.

The merlin was passed on to a friend who is a knowledgeable ornithologist with a large flight aviary. There our patient gained strength at an amazing pace. One day when the aviary door was opened at feeding time the merlin made his break for freedom. Like a bullet he hit the narrow gap through the part-open door.

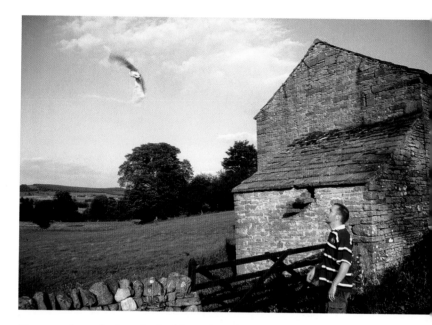

He was released where he had been found, and made a bee-line for a favourite perch in a big sycamore.

And then something amazing happened. Perhaps he was just finding his bearings, but he soared, twisted, turned, and showed off his flying skills for a full two minutes as if to announce, "I'll be fine," and "Thanks for your attention."

Being a vet has many magic moments, but well up the list comes successful treatment of our feathered friends and launching them back into the air.

25 . . . and a Partridge on a Stone Wall

I've long been fascinated by the thousands of miles of dry-stone walls in the Pennines. They flanked my route throughout my travels in the dale, and they provide the stitching in the patchwork quilt of fields which form the broad panorama of the dales landscape.

The walls look as though they have been there for ever, but most were constructed in about forty years at the turn of the eighteenth/nineteenth century when the Enclosure Acts came into force. At a ton of stone to every yard of wall, this represents quite a flurry of building activity. In the Yorkshire Dales alone, it is estimated that there are five thousand miles of wall. That equates to almost nine million tons, with each stone placed individually by craftsmen's hands. The total weight for the whole of the Pennines must be astronomical.

The structure is that of a three-dimensional jigsaw, with every stone counterbalancing the next so that no mortar is necessary. The random crevices so produced have led to further fascination, for they are, to anyone like me with a keen interest in natural history, an Aladdin's cave.

Over the next couple of hundred years the walls were colonised by all manner of wildlife. Amphibians, reptiles, small mammals and birds all took advantage of this new facility, some making their homes there. Mosses, ferns, grasses, and flowering plants turned the wall into a botanists' paradise.

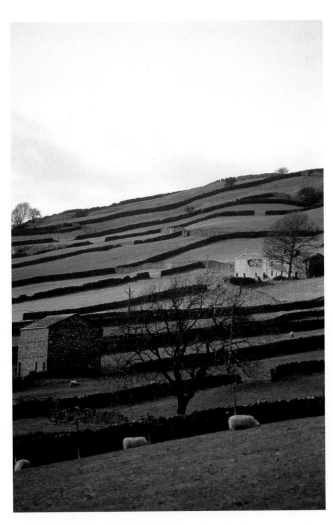

Ranks of stone walls across the dales landscape

The most successful colonists are lichens. Everywhere there are crusts, scales, plaques, and shrubby little growths. Most people never give them a second glance, but the story of the lichen truly is a bizarre tale, for the lichen is not just one plant. It's a fungus and a microscopic alga living together in symbiosis, to their mutual advantage. The fungus provides shelter and a water-retentive environment for the alga, while the alga synthesises nutrients, which it shares with the fungus. The alga is capable of living, and often does, a totally independent lifestyle. It can produce all its necessities of life from raw materials, but the fungus cannot. Without its algal partner, the fungus would die.

Frogs and toads use ponds in the breeding season, but spend most of the rest of the year on land. A damp niche at the foot of a dry-stone wall is a favourite spot.

Reptiles are cold blooded and need to warm up before any vigorous activity. The walls act like storage heaters, and I would regularly see lizards basking on tops of the walls. Slow worms and adders would snuggle up to the base of the wall to soak up the radiated heat.

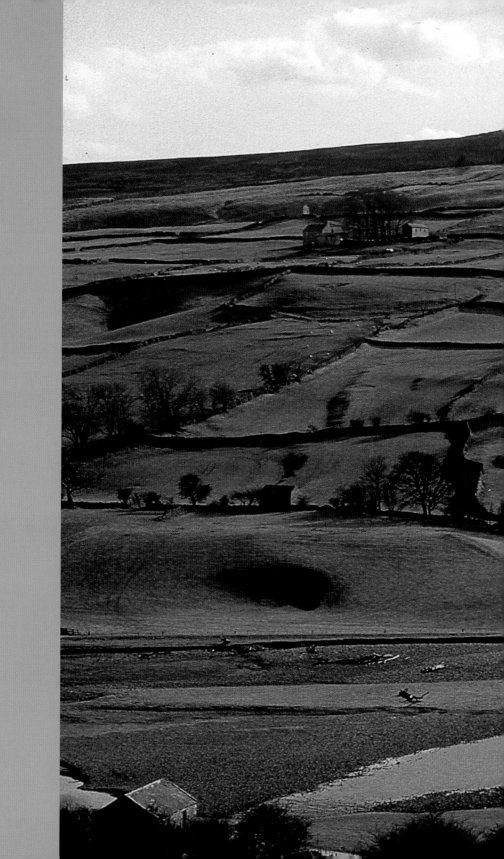

Stone walls form a patchwork quilt above the river.

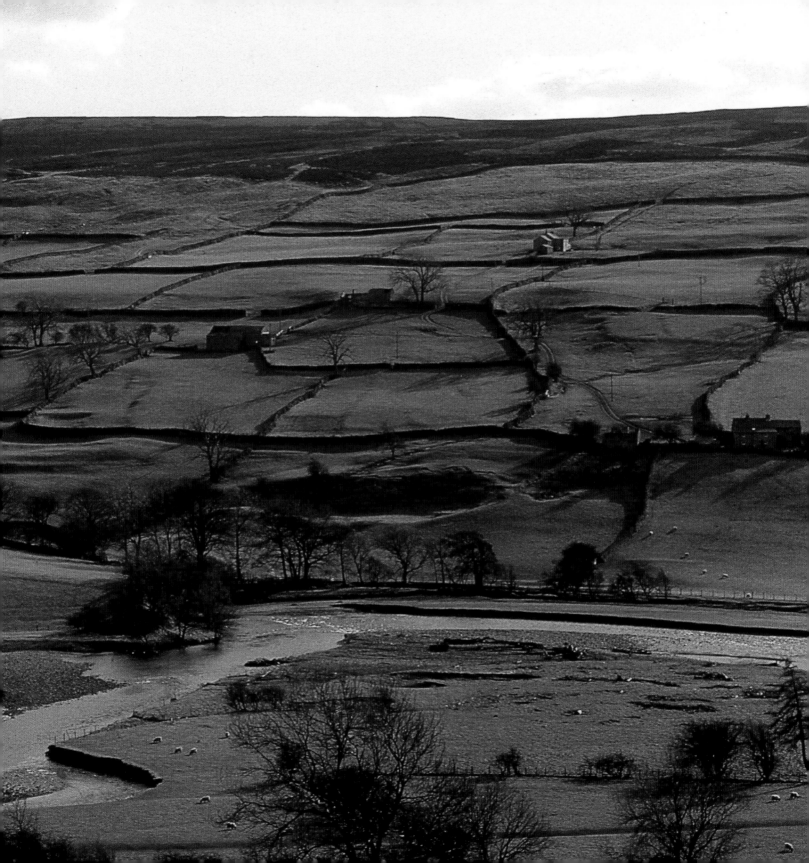

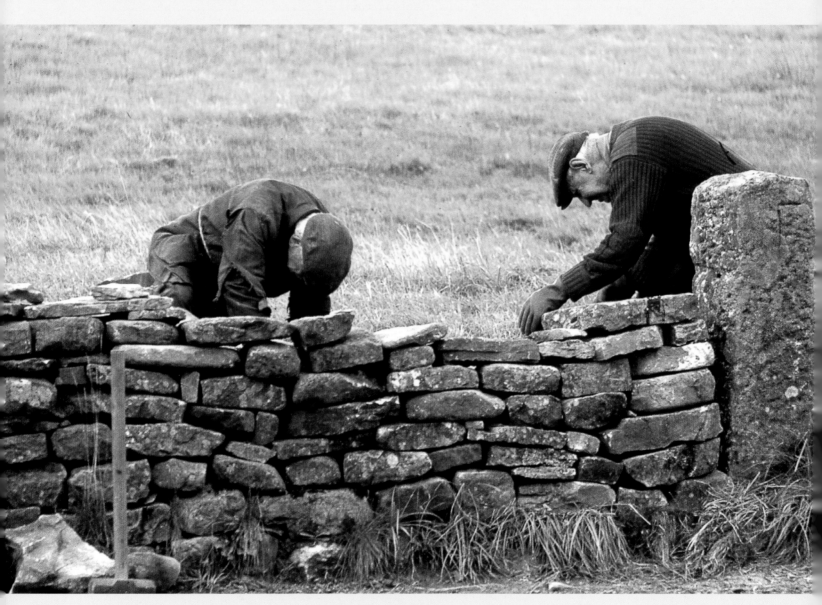

Most farmers are quite skilled at repairing gaps in the walls.

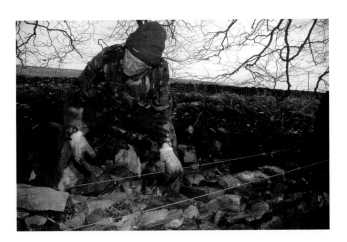

Ken is a full-time stone-waller. He has a great knowledge of the countryside, and if I had time I would stop and have a chat. He told me the story of how he had saved the life of a slow worm by building it some winter quarters.

A friend of mine, Ken, is a full-time professional waller, and he tells a wonderful story of an encounter with a slow worm.

In the depths of winter he was repairing a stone wall and inadvertently exposed a hibernating slow worm. Concerned for its welfare, he found a bucket, half filled it with soil, and topped it with stones to create a grotto for the sleepy creature. He took the bucket home and kept it in his shed till spring, then at the first signs of waking he took the little reptile back to exactly where he had found it.

He was thrilled to see it snake its way back into the crevices of the wall.

All manner of birds, both wild and domestic, use the top of the wall as a vantage point, either to announce their presence, or to have a good look around. Having an interest in photography, it became a passion of mine to capture a selection of "wall-top" portraits. A handsome bird with a background of blue sky is a very attractive composition.

In the winter the dale can be the bleakest of places, but the return of the waders in the spring is an exciting time. Their aerial displays and calls announce the end of winter. Curlews, redshanks, and oystercatchers are great posers. They love to sit on the wall top to announce their arrival. But they are also very shy.

The only chance of setting up the perfect portrait comes in June when their eggs have hatched, and they anxiously shepherd and guard their precious chicks. Only then will they hold their ground and use an elevated position to keep an eye on their young and to assess the threat from the intruder with the telephoto lens pointing out of the car window.

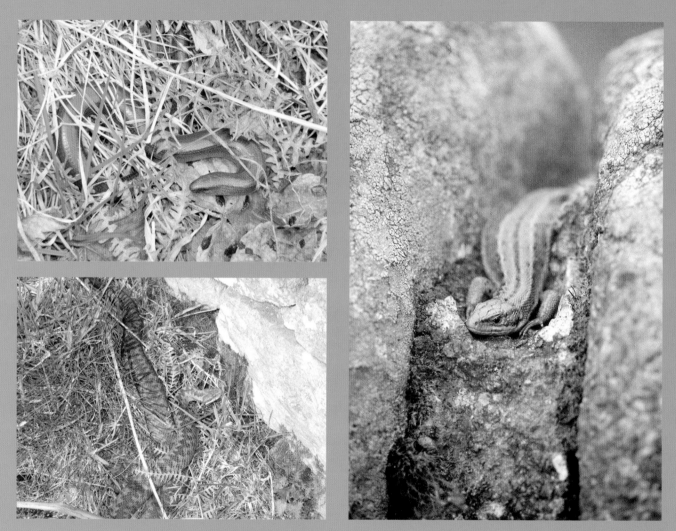

Reptiles are cold blooded, and since the walls act like storage heaters, they will bask in the radiated heat to warm themselves up. Here we see a slow worm, an adder, and a common lizard.

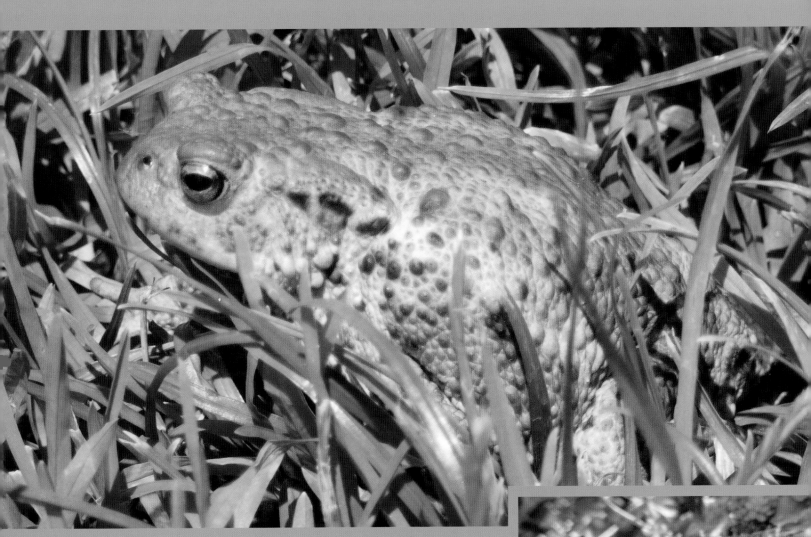

Frogs and toads like to find damp niches at the foot of stone walls.

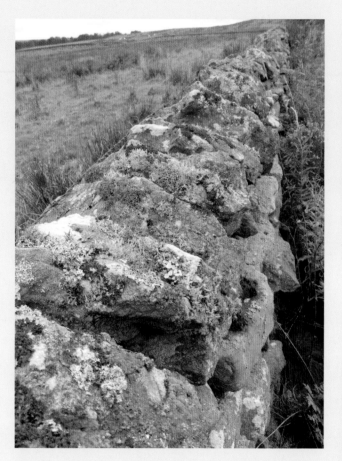

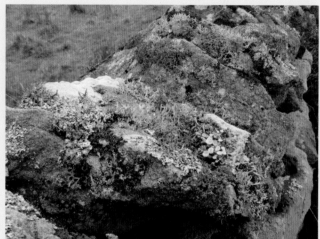

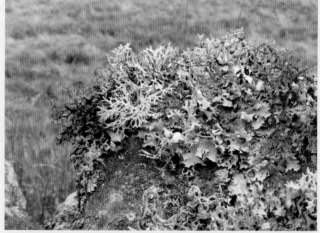

Lichens flourish on stone walls. They cannot tolerate atmospheric pollution, which would suggest that the pure dales air is to their liking.

Partridge are never seen at wall-top level. They spend almost their whole life at ground level, keeping a low profile. Their defence mechanism, should danger threaten, is to simply "freeze" into immobility. Ground vegetation usually provides excellent camouflage, and they become instantly invisible.

However, one day as I drove down a typical dales country road I spotted a partridge perched on the top of the wall ahead of me.

Instead of flying away or hopping down to ground level, something triggered its "sit-tight" reflex. And there he was, four and a half feet off the ground, locked in his instinctive posture, fondly imagining that he was invisible. I stopped the car next to the bird and hurriedly took a few pictures but he stayed transfixed. I wondered if, at some point, he would discover that he was perched on the wall for all to see, but he remained convinced that he was invisible.

Eventually I returned to the car and drove on, bemused that the partridge was, at that moment, congratulating himself on the success of his camouflage!

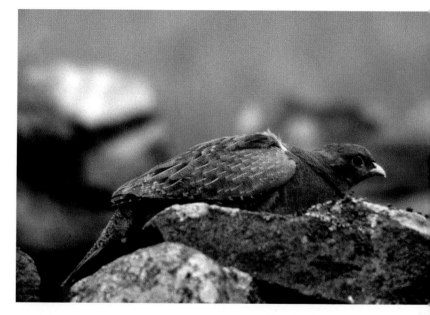

The "partridge on a stone wall".

My approach triggered his instinctive defence mechanism, which was to freeze into immobility. At ground level this is a good strategy. On top of a wall it's not such a good idea, but he was convinced that he was invisible.

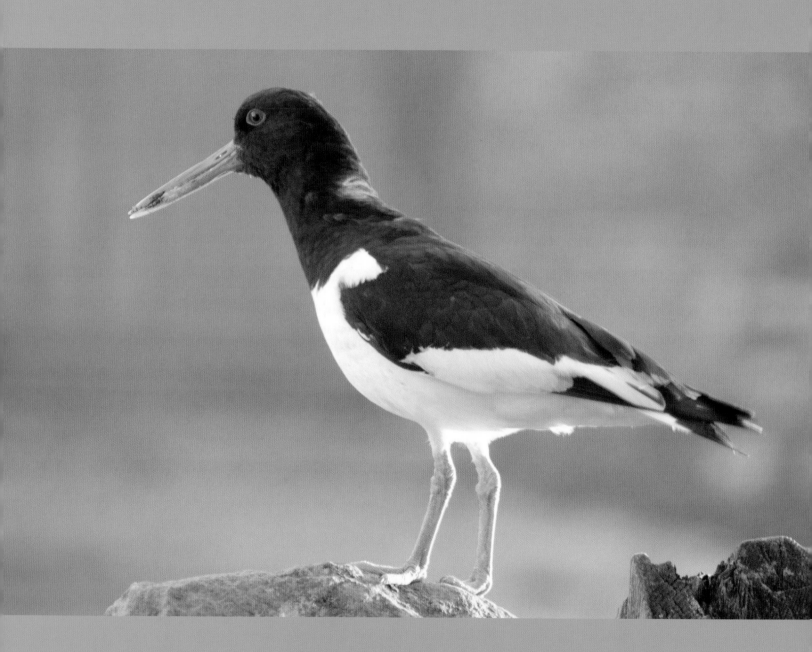

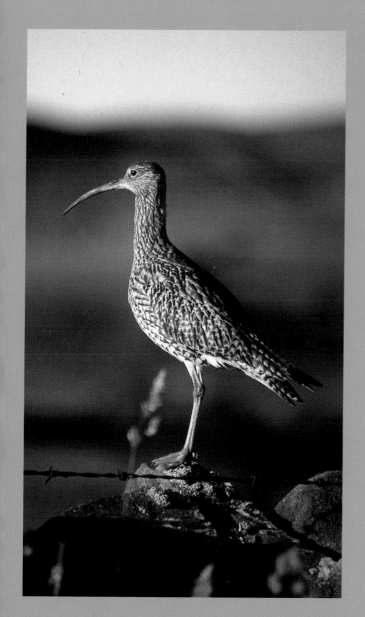

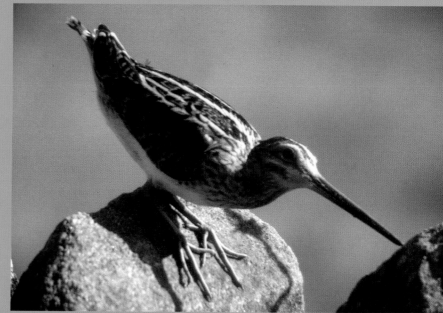

The wading birds like to perch on wall tops. Here we see an oystercatcher, curlew, and a snipe.

26 The Ancient Mysteries of the Felon

S oon after I first came to the dales in 1973 a client summoned me to a case of "felon". I'd never heard the word before, but didn't care to confess my ignorance. The old dales farmer on the other end of the phone would have thought that this young vet didn't know much if I'd asked what it was!

When I arrived at the farm and examined the animal, it turned out to be a case of summer mastitis, a condition with which I was fully familiar. But the term "felon" intrigued me, for it was frequently used by the older dales farmers in many contexts. The *Oxford English Dictionary* threw some light on the subject, for it was described as an archaic term meaning an acute inflammatory swelling. My client had used the term correctly, for summer mastitis is, indeed, an acute inflammatory swelling of the udder. This mediaeval term had survived in the dalesman's vocabulary for hundreds of years.

In another context I had heard that the old "cow doctors" would perform a surgical procedure called "cutting for felon". A cut would be made in a loose flap of skin between the forelegs of a cow, and a small bundle of "felon grass" would be inserted into the wound. Left there for a few days the irritant juices of this foreign body would provoke a violent inflammatory response.

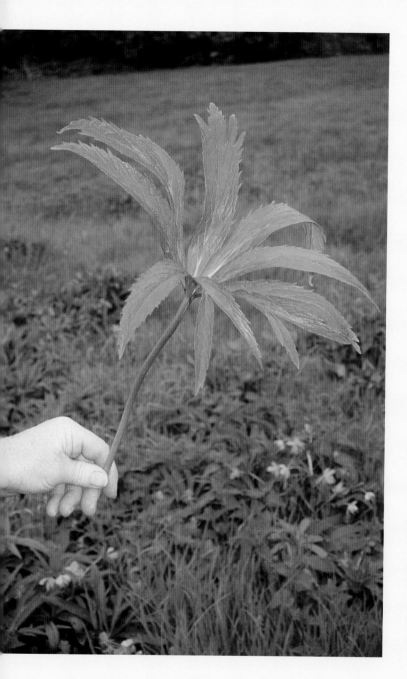

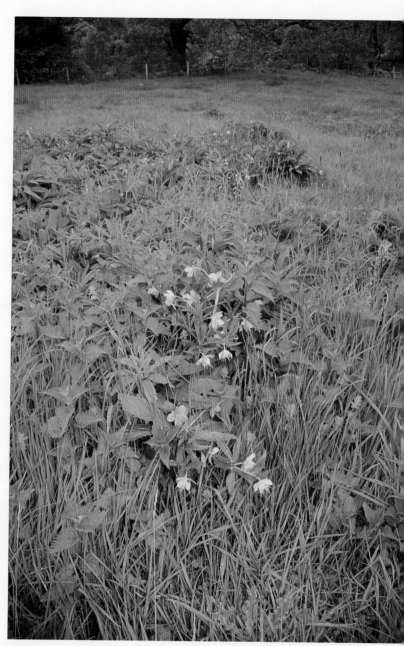

Helleborus viridis, the "felon grass".

The procedure was used on cattle that were in poor condition. Apparently the "poor doer" immediately began to thrive. However, I suspect that once the ailing individual was identified and treated, it received better care and feeding, which probably accounted for the success of the treatment. Some of my older clients had actually seen the operation performed when they were youngsters.

I had thought that "cutting for felon" was very much a dales tradition, but a veterinary colleague told me that when he was working in Somerset he had heard of a similar practice being carried out in the old days. In the Somerset version, copper wire was inserted into the wound. He added that the Voortrekkers in South Africa used to carry out a similar procedure, but used the skin of the tail as opposed to the dewlap.

The identity of the plant referred to as felon grass eluded me for many years. Eventually, by speaking with friends and clients who had an interest in local folklore, I learned that it was not a grass, but a hellebore, Helleborus viridis. The plant is quite rare in the north of England but was said to grow in two or three sites in the dale. My next task was to track it down.

When at last I found the felon grass, it added to the mystery of my quest, for it seemed to be growing in a neat rectangular patch in the middle of a large field. It was as though it had been purposely cultivated as a monoculture in a walled garden, and the walls had disappeared as if by magic!

In *Gerard's Herbal*, published in 1597, he tells us of Helleborus that

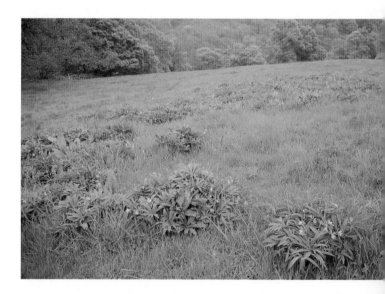

This picture shows the rectangular patch in the middle of a field. One could imagine that it had been cultivated in the borders of a walled garden, and that the walls had mysteriously disappeared.

it be good against the falling sicknesse, phrensies, sciatica, dropsies, poison, and against all cold diseases which be of hard curation, and will not yield to any gentle medicine. The poudre drawne up the nose causeth sneesing, and purgeth the brain from grosse and slimy humours.

He does, however, recommend caution, saying,

This strong medicine ought not to be given inwardly to delicate bodies, but it may be more safely given unto countrey people which feed grossly, and have hard, tough, and strong bodies.

It would seem that it's OK for hardy dales folk!

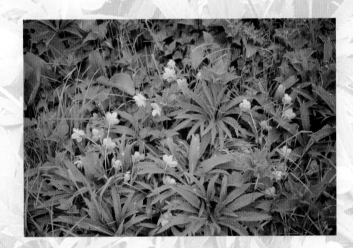

27 A Big Splash of Yellow

One of the exciting aspects of my working life was a day-to-day intimacy with the dales landscape. With such familiarity it was easy to observe changes, be they subtle or dramatic, taking place.

For instance there are three occasions in the year when Mother Nature dips a large paintbrush into a big pot of yellow paint and splashes it generously across vast swathes of the dales landscape.

The first occurs in March, and although it is quite widespread, it seems to be most evident in the dales churchyards. It is caused by millions of celandines bursting into bloom.

The second splash is much more noticeable, occurring on a grand scale in the traditional hay meadows and pastures of the upper dale. Dales winters are usually incredibly wet. Huge quantities of rain are deposited as the Atlantic westerlies hit the high Pennines, and the land soaks it up till it can soak up no more. In spring the boggy fields are ideal for the marsh marigold. They flourish there. Throughout April the glossy leaves form a wall-to-wall carpet in the fields, then in early May there is an explosion of vibrant yellow flower heads. It makes one wonder how this bog garden, in a few weeks, will turn into a dales hay meadow, but it does.

The third splash is rather special. Again it happens in the traditionally managed hay meadows in the upper dale.

The globeflower (Trollius europaeus) is one of the most spectacular flowers in the dales. It seems to have its favourite meadows, where swathes of yellow colour the landscape in June and July. Apart from its great beauty, it's a fascinating subject for the naturalist. A drama that is carried out every summer inside its tightly closed flower head is a lesson on how nature has designed subtle, but incredibly complicated relationships between many of its species.

The spectacular globeflower is just that—a globe, which never actually opens fully like most familiar flowers. This, you would think, would exclude pollinating insects which are vital to reproduction and survival of the species.

And in a way, you'd be right.

However, whilst most insects just can't get in, nature has evolved half a dozen specialist species of a small fly called chiastocheta, which are expert at entering the globe to access pollen and nectar. Scientists have identified sixteen scents secreted by Trollius, and six of these are irresistible to chiastocheta.

So far, so good.

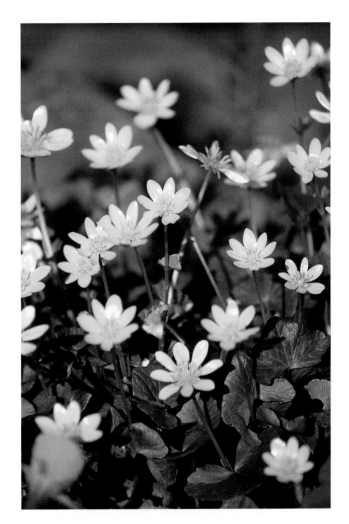

Celandines in a dales churchyard.

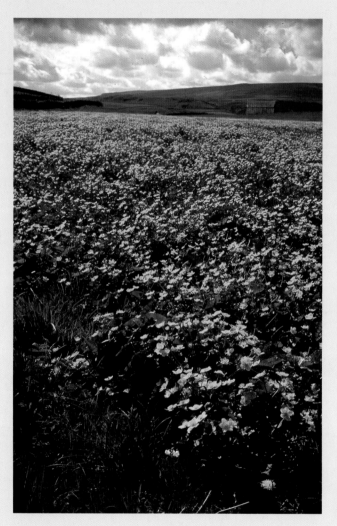

Marsh marigolds painting the dales landscape in yellow.

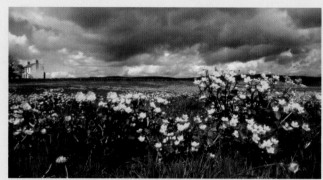

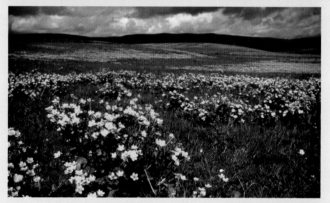

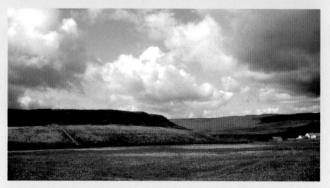

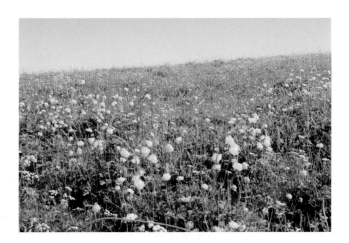

Globeflowers seem to have their favourite hay meadows. Some fields have none, but in others, like this one, they flourish in huge numbers.

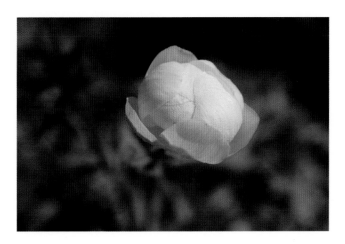

Its name describes its form perfectly. It's a compact globe.

Now for the bad news. Chiastocheta, having been attracted to the irresistible scents, lays its eggs inside the flower, and the fly larvae like nothing better than munching on the developing seeds there. In fact they eat nothing else, and if they were to eat all the seeds there would be none left to ensure globeflowers next summer, nor any summer after that. This is not just bad news for the globeflower, it's bad news for the fly, for if the globeflower died out, the very specialised chiastocheta would rapidly follow.

Nature, however, has thought of that, and has taken steps to keep the fly and the flower happy. The more munching of seeds that goes on, the more the flower is stimulated to produce a flavonoid chemical called adonivernith, which limits larval growth and feeding. Thus the number of successful larvae is contained, and a satisfactory amount of seeds will survive to germinate next year.

Isn't nature very clever?

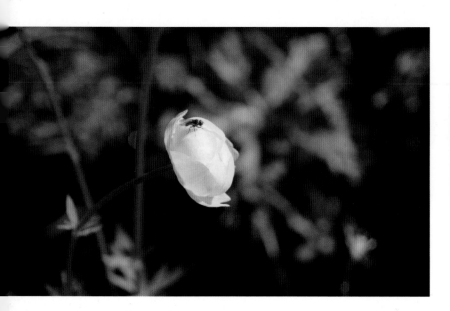

Chiastocheta arrives.

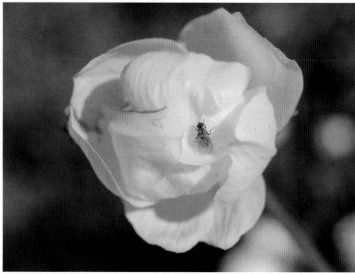

If you look closely you'll see pollen grains sticking to the hairs on the fly's back.

28 The Magic Sponge

David Bellamy, famous botanist and conservationist, once described the tops of the Pennine hills as "a great big mossy sponge".

The Atlantic westerlies sweep in from the ocean, and once they hit the high Pennines they dump enormous quantities of rain. The peaty, mossy landscape soaks it all up, and then gradually releases it to form rivulets. These rivulets ooze from the earth and coalesce to form little streams. The streams are referred to as "becks" in this part of the world, one of many relics of the Old Norse that punctuates the northern vocabulary.

The becks, in turn, coalesce to form minor rivers, which are the tributaries of the great rivers that flow from the Pennines to the North Sea. Tyne, Wear, and

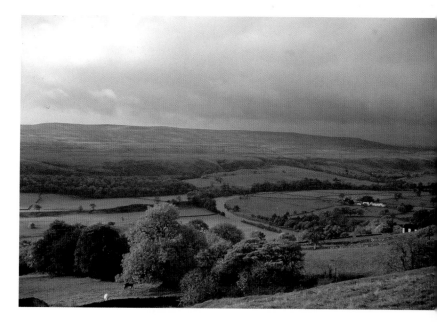

An Atlantic westerly rolls in to drop huge amounts of water on the already saturated "big mossy sponge".

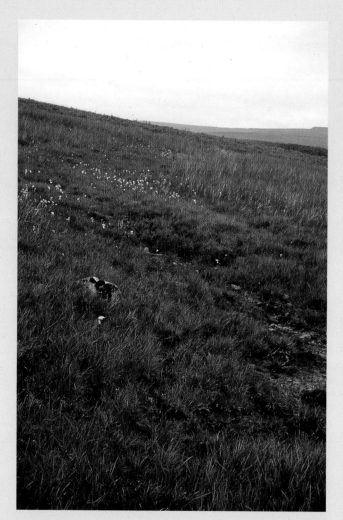
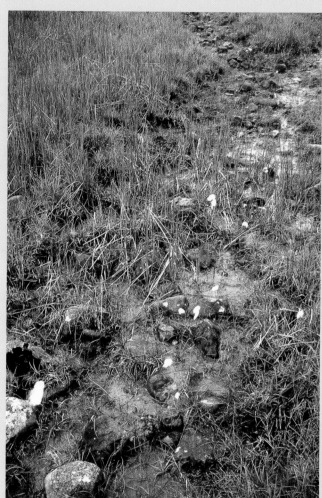

The whole landscape oozes rivulets which flow into the becks.

Tees flow directly to the sea, while Swale, Wharfe, Ure, Aire, Nidd, Calder, and Don all join up to form the Yorkshire Ouse. Over the millennia, their flow has carved great chasms in the carboniferous rock, and given us the landscape that we now refer to as "The Dales".

The becks, too, in their downhill rush have created steep-sided little valleys. These are referred to as "gills", again from the Old Norse. On the west of the great Pennine watershed, and particularly in the Lake District, the word assumes the more picturesque spelling of "ghyll", but the pronunciation is the same.

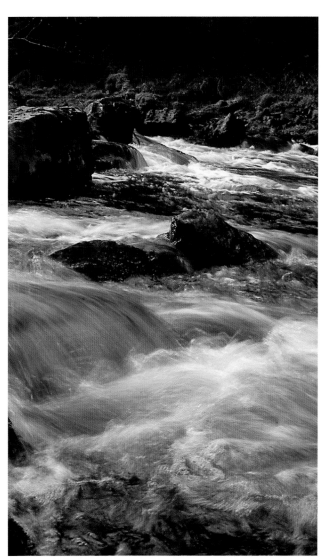

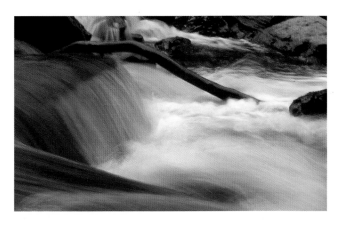

The peaty waters of the beck.

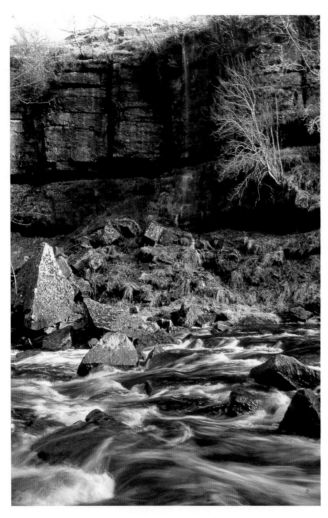

Here you see a little waterfall oozing from the moor to swell the Sleightholme Beck.

Occasionally a cow would stumble into a gill, roll down the precipitous embankment, and embed itself in the mire below. The vet was usually called upon to supervise the rescue operation, and it was always a very physical, hands-on manoeuvre. It was necessary to summon as many sturdy neighbours as possible to do the heaving. However, I'd be at the sharp end tying the ropes and trying to control the stressed patient thrashing about in the mire. Once the patient was on her feet I would lead her down the stream bed till more level ground was reached. It must have been quite a sight to see cow and vet, bedraggled and exhausted, emerging triumphant but soaked to the skin and caked in a coating of peaty mud. "The Monsters from the Black Lagoon" would have been an apt caption.

Each gill seems to have its own character. In the upper dale they can be stark and almost treeless, with an expanse of rushy bog in the bottom. Further east their character changes, as rivulets tumble over exposed rocks in bubbling cascades. Rowan, hazel, and alder form a guard of honour as the water makes its way to the great river below.

Still further down the dale the character changes again. Ancient conifers abound. Ferns, mosses and lichens festoon the low branches of the trees, imparting a mystical aura. In the spring, primroses punctuate the vivid greens of the ground vegetation, and, as summer progresses, the air is filled with the aroma of wild garlic. It is the stuff of Arthurian legend.

Throughout the length of the gills there is a constant reminder that we are still in the "big mossy sponge". A continuous flow of water oozes over the rim of the gill. Drips, trickles, and picturesque cascades swell the volume of the stream below.

The sheer volume of the squeezings from the landscape is not obvious until spells in winter when severe frosts occur. The oozing water solidifies to form gigantic icicles. Some years ago my wife, Chris, and I came upon this phenomenon quite by chance.

An injured tawny owl had been brought to us for medical attention. The damage wasn't too serious. It had probably sustained a glancing blow on the head from a passing motor car and was concussed. Treatment in these cases is straightforward, and almost always successful. For the first few days the bird is kept warm and quiet. As soon as the bird is feeding well and flying around the aviary it is released.

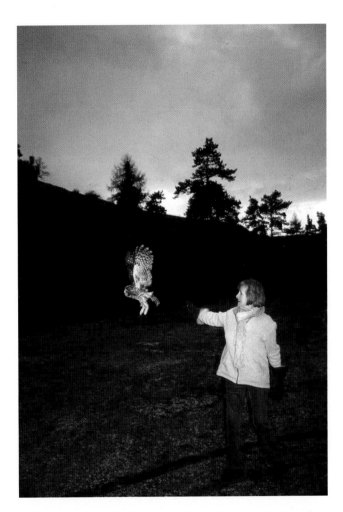

It was in a gill that we released one of our patients. Light was fading and we suspected that sub-zero temperatures over the previous week had given rise to some pretty ice formations. We resolved to return the next day to see them.

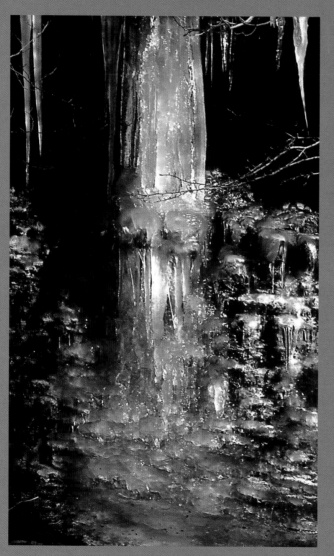
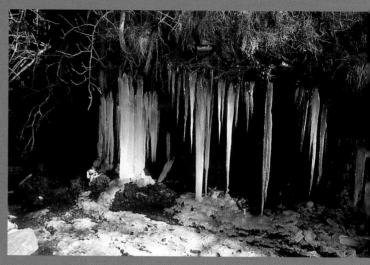
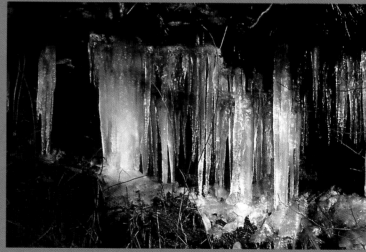

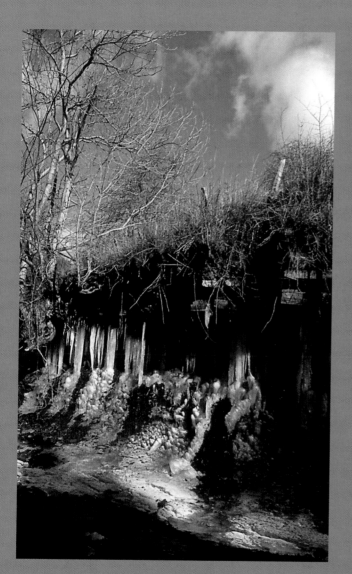

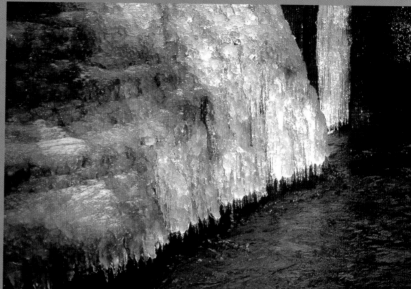

Vast quantities of water oozing from the landscape had transformed the gill into a spectacular ice palace.

Since owls are territorial, we try to release the bird as soon as possible and as near as possible to the place where it was found. It is also quite important to release the patient at dusk to avoid it being mobbed by day-flying birds. The owl had been found in a gill, and as we took our patient to its point of release in a clearing on the banks of the stream we were astounded at the sight. Although the light was fading, we could see that a series of hard frosts had been at work on the ooze from the big mossy sponge. The little valley had been transformed into something like an ice palace from a fairy story.

We released the owl (we still feel a thrill of achievement at the conclusion of every successful case) and resolved to return the following day to investigate more of nature's ice sculptures on the banks of the gill.

The next day Chris and I had a memorable walk along the banks of the stream. A strong, low, winter sun set the sheets of ice and the ranks of icicles twinkling. It was a revelation, and another reason to admire the wonders of the Pennine gills.

29 Fodder and Fieldhouses

I once happened to arrive in a farmyard at exactly the same time as an awesome convoy.

A large yellow piece of agricultural machinery resembling a combine harvester led the column. In its wake followed three gigantic blue tractors, each pulling a bright red trailer the size of a railway goods van. The flamboyant colours and the deafening throb of the engines were, as I said, awesome.

I made my way to the relative quiet of the cattle accommodation where the farmer and his ailing cow waited. The examination was time consuming, and the treatment was complicated, but I completed my work in about half an hour, said my farewells, and returned to the car. On the way I was greeted by an amazing sight.

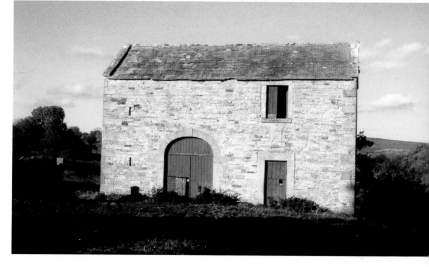

All fieldhouses are different, but they are all similar in that they have a hayloft above, and a cow byre at ground level. The large door allows a trailer to be backed in, and hay forked into the hayloft.

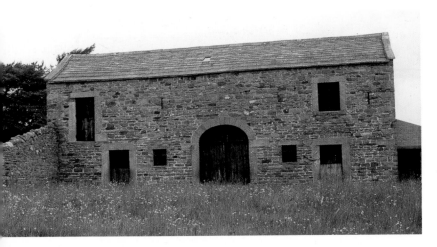

A bigger fieldhouse with two byres.

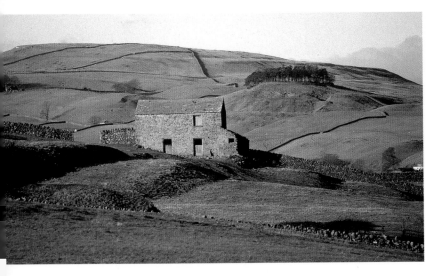

Some fieldhouses were built on a hillside to facilitate heaving hay from ground level into the loft with a pitchfork.

While I had been attending my patient, the awesome convoy had sprung into action. The better part of a huge field of grass had been lifted, chopped, and deposited in the silage clamp with clinical efficiency. Within minutes, a significant proportion of the herd's winter rations had been secured. This was high-tech farming.

I could not help but wonder at the dramatic changes that had taken place in just a few decades. For centuries, most farms in the dales had used the "fieldhouse" system, the fieldhouse being a stone barn with a hayloft above and a cow byre below. There must be thousands of these buildings scattered around the Pennine meadows, and every one is different. Planners and designers played no part in their solid, enduring construction. Common sense and function were the defining factors.

Fieldhouses were always situated in hay meadows where, in summer, the grass would be cut, dried, and transported to the hayloft. When the cattle returned from the high pastures in autumn they would graze the late growth on the meadows before being housed in the fieldhouse for the winter. Tranches of hay in the loft could be cut away and dropped through a trapdoor to the byre below, and fed to the cattle.

Throughout the winter, manure was transferred to the dung heap or "midden" outside, and in the spring, when the cattle were turned out to the high pastures, it was spread on the meadow to ensure a good hay crop in the summer.

Before the advent of the internal combustion engine, all of this was accomplished by manpower and horsepower. The grass was cut by ranks of men with scythes. Turning, spreading, and rowing up took hours of painstaking work with the hay rake. A spell of rain at the wrong moment meant that the process would have to be repeated. Having been satisfactorily dried, horse-drawn "sweeps" would then drag piles of hay to the fieldhouse where it

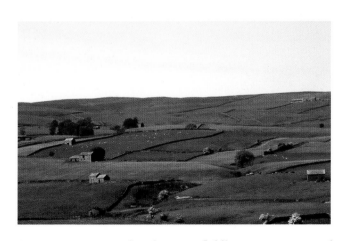

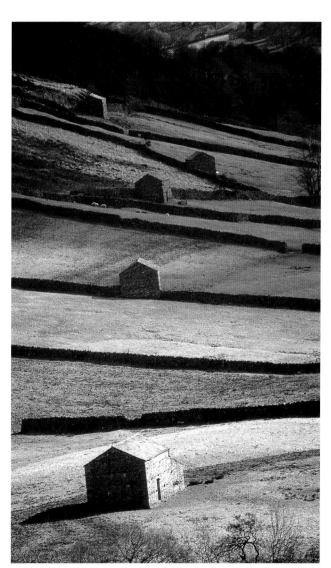

Sometimes it seems that there is a fieldhouse in every meadow.

was launched into the hayloft by stout men with pitchforks.

The whole family plus neighbours and friends would commit to hours of hard work in the hayfield. There wasn't time for them to return to the farmhouse for meals, so meals were brought to the hayfield. Although the system was labour intensive by today's standards, the practicality

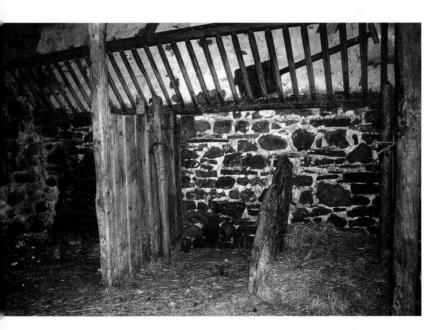

A traditional interior with wooden double stalls and a wooden hayrack. Each double stall is divided by a large slab of stone, most of which is buried in the ground.

was admirable and the fieldhouse system was an eminently simple strategy in dales farming. However, with the advancing mechanisation of the mid twentieth century, and the practice of baling hay, one man on a tractor could now accomplish all the tasks that once had occupied a huge workforce.

It was in an old fieldhouse that I faced one of my most spectacular near-death experiences. The farmer, his farmhand, and I walked to a fieldhouse, where, in order to conduct my examination, I needed to squeeze between my patient and her neighbour in a double stall. Both had seemed docile until I was in position, but then one of the cows panicked, and this spooked her neighbour.

Suddenly, there was I, sandwiched between two demented cows. All hell had let loose. Both were striking at me from both ends. Well-aimed kicks from their hind feet hammered into my thighs, while their heads were intent on butting me into oblivion.

Adrenalin must have taken over, for I felt no pain. I was able to observe calmly that there was no way out of this predicament. I was aware only of the importance of staying upright. I knew that if I lost my footing it would be the end. The crazed animals

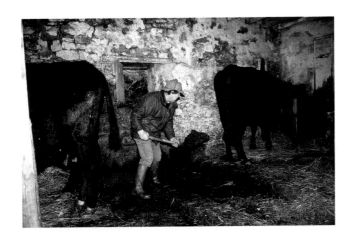

Many fieldhouses have a dung channel sloping to one end of the building. Dung can be pushed to the wall at the bottom end and delivered to the dung heap or "midden" through a hole in the wall.

would kick and stamp until every bone in my body was broken.

And then something touched my head. It was a rope. The two men had realised that there was no escape at ground level, but had noticed that I was directly under the trapdoor that was used to drop hay to the byre below. They had scurried up to the hayloft, then lowered a rope, and hauled me to safety.

As life threatening as it had been, the scenario of a young vet swinging through the air like a pantomime Peter Pan in wellies has to have its funny side.

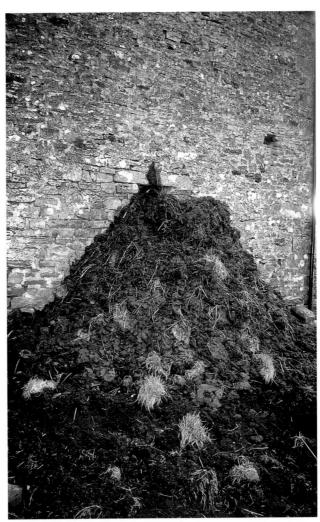

The muck heap. This will be spread on the meadows in the spring to ensure a good hay crop. If you look carefully you'll see an airborne shovelful on its way to the midden.

Sadly nowadays the fieldhouses are becoming redundant. Many are falling into disrepair, although a few have been tastefully converted into homes of character. They do, however, remain an integral part of the dales landscape.

Massive new buildings have been erected close to the farmsteads. Whole herds can be accommodated under one roof. Winter rations are stored nearby and dispensed by high-tech machinery. No longer is the spectre of a disastrous hay crop a nightmare for the dales farmer. No longer does he have to see his stock barely surviving winter on a diet of blackened, fungus-ridden hay after a wet summer.

The awesome convoy has seen to that.

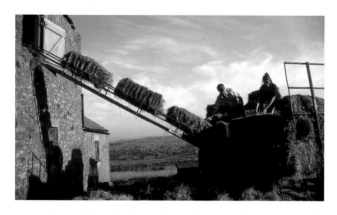

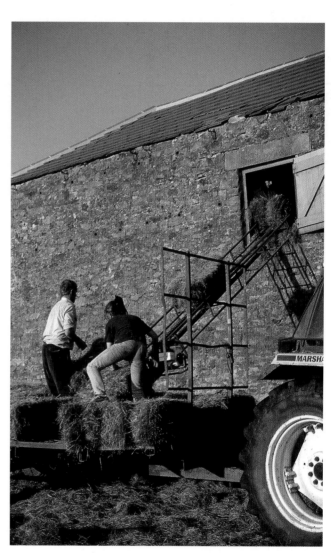

Loose hay used to be heaved into the hayloft with pitchforks. This was superceded by hay bales and a petrol-driven elevator. Big bales have now largely replaced these small bales.

30 The Hay Meadows of the High Pennines

I marvel at the natural beauty of the dales. Yet, strictly speaking, it is not a natural landscape at all. Man created it, and if it were not maintained by man, nature would take over and it would quickly revert to primaeval forest. Most of northern Europe was densely forested until man arrived.

At the end of the last Ice Age, twelve thousand years ago, the glaciers retreated and left a tundra-like landscape which was subsequently colonised by birch, hazel, pine, oak, and elm. For much of that time birch was the dominant species.

Six thousand years ago Stone Age hunter-gatherers arrived in this wooded landscape, home to wild boar, auroch, wolf, elk, and lynx. These people cleared areas of woodland to create small farmsteads. Gradually the hunter-gatherers changed their lifestyle and became farmers.

By the Iron Age, little of the wooded landscape remained. The clearances continued, and were so complete that virtually none of it survives today, although in the upper dale we do have one of the best examples of the relic birch forest, at Park End Wood.

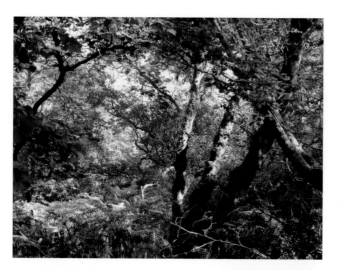

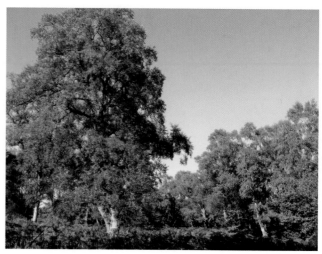

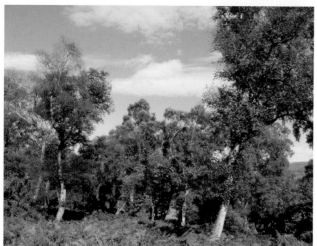

Primaeval birch forest, much as it was when Neolithic man arrived in the dale six thousand years ago. Man removed the trees to change his lifestyle from hunter-gatherer to farmer. By the Iron Age there was very little forest left.

In the newly formed grassland a diverse flora evolved. It became a unique ecosystem. Up to 120 different botanical species occur in some of the richer meadows. Mother Nature, as is her wont, designed a clever balance. Semi-parasitic plants such as yellow rattle and eyebright kept rampant grass growth in check, allowing the diverse flora to flourish. The climate dictated that haymaking seldom began before the end of July, by which time seed had been set, ensuring continuity of the species the following year.

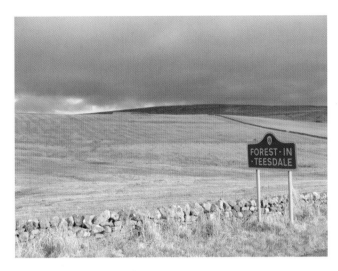

It's ironic that there is a parish at the top of the dale called Forest-in-Teesdale, and there's not a tree in sight.

whole meadows were ploughed up, reseeded with a monoculture of more productive grasses, and managed intensively.

As a result the species-rich ecosystem of the traditional hay meadow went into decline. In just a few decades, ninety-eight per cent disappeared, until, in May 2006, the North Pennines Area of Outstanding Natural Beauty (AONB) Partnership initiated the "Hay Time" project with the remit to protect the surviving meadows and to restore and enhance at least 140 hectares of upland hay meadows to bring the total in the North Pennines

This spectacular feature of the landscape endured for two thousand years.

However, pressures of modern agriculture in the mid twentieth century led to sweeping changes in farming practices. Meadows that had been managed to produce a modest crop of hay, abetted only by a modest application of "farmyard manure" in the spring, began to disappear.

Many fields were encouraged to produce huge crops of winter fodder by liberal application of nitrogen-based fertilisers. In more extreme cases,

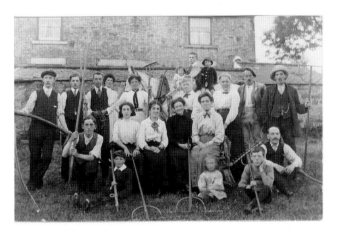

A hundred years ago haymaking was very labour intensive. Family, neighbours, and friends were needed to share the heavy workload.

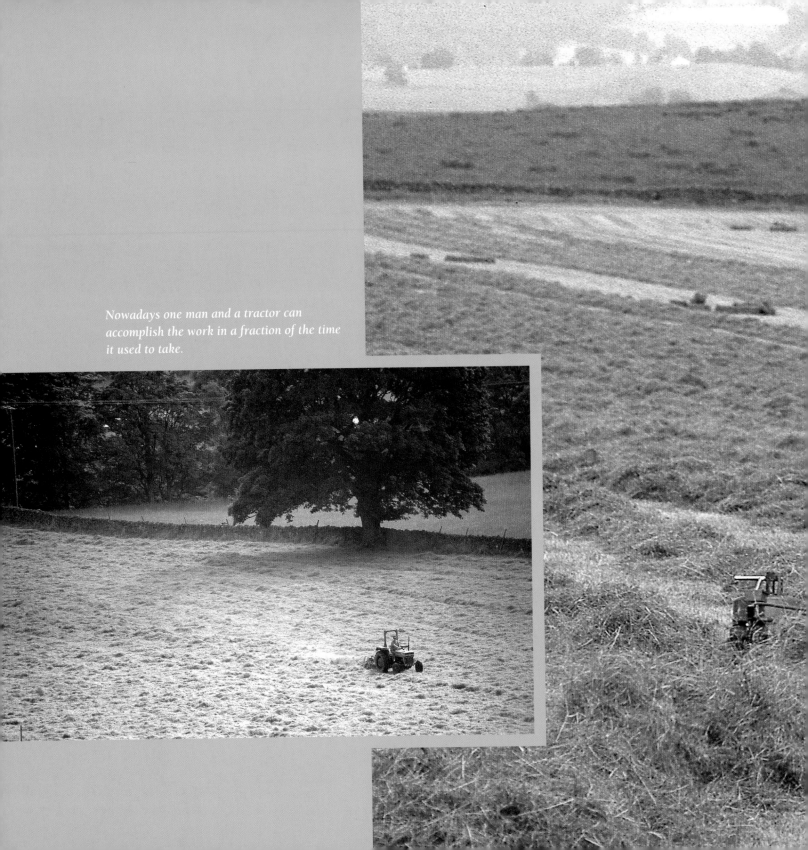

Nowadays one man and a tractor can accomplish the work in a fraction of the time it used to take.

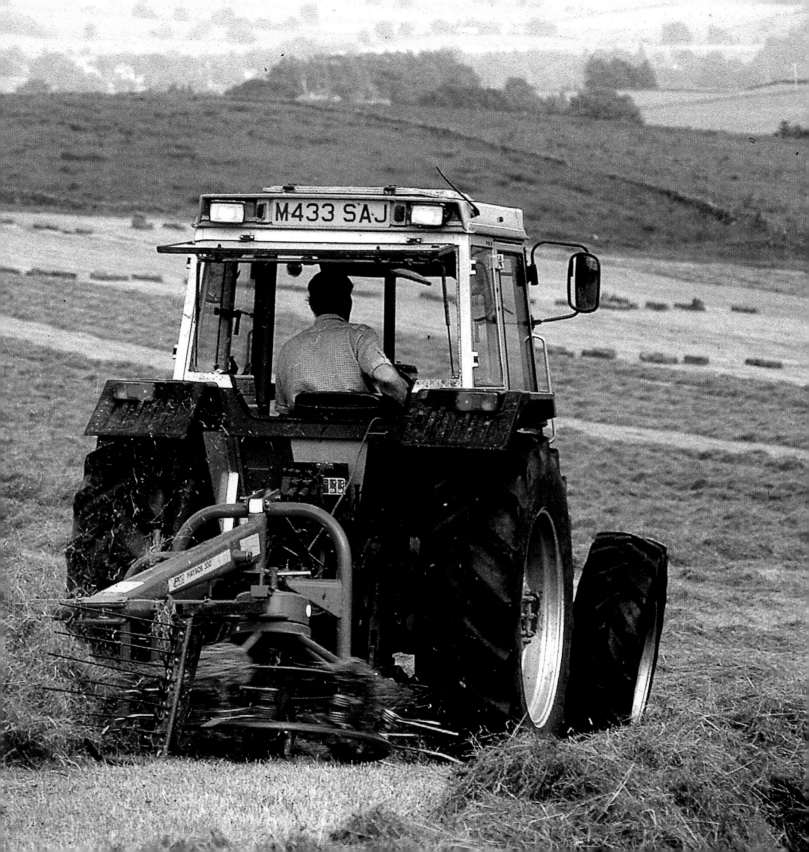

to over 500 hectares. At the same time it aimed to "increase people's awareness, enjoyment and understanding of this important habitat".

A limited amount of meadow that was under intensive management has been earmarked for regeneration. Seeded grass and flowers in a species-rich traditional meadow are cut and collected. This is transferred to a muck-spreader, which transports the seeded grass and scatters it on a meadow that has been scarified to ensure the new seeds find a niche. To further increase chances of success, cattle are introduced to the field. Their feet push the seed further into the sward to favour germination.

As part of the project, I was commissioned to document, in pictures, a year in the life of a traditional hay meadow.

I travelled 1700 miles, spent 120 hours "in the field", sat for about 300 hours in front of a computer screen, and amassed a library of about 5000 images.

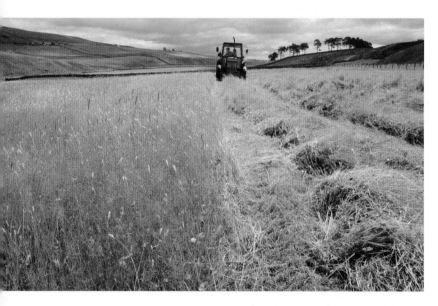

Cutting a traditional hay meadow. Note the many different grasses present.

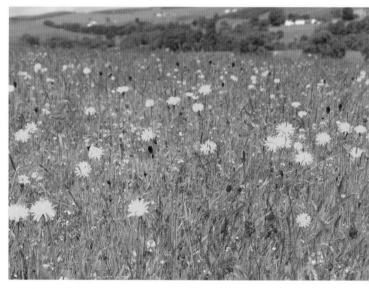

A traditional hay meadow, which can hold up to 120 different botanical species.

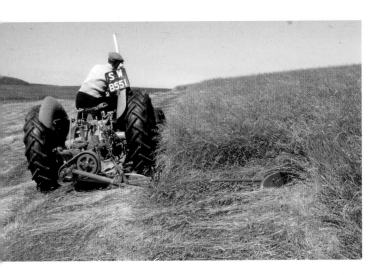

In the 1950s some meadows were ploughed, seeded with a monoculture of productive grass, and treated with artificial fertiliser. This was one of the first to use this system in the dale. Note that there is only one species of grass and there are no flowers at all.

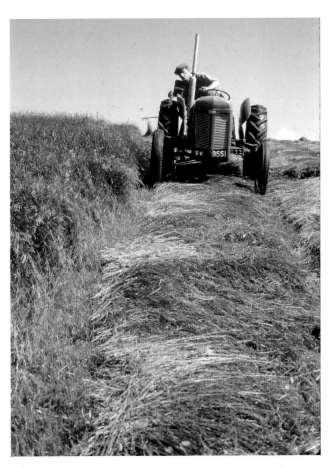

It was hard work, but an absolute joy. So much more was added to my knowledge of the natural history of these magical places. The result was an exhibition of photographs which toured the north for seven weeks, stimulating an awareness of the importance of this gem of the British countryside.

My friends, the hill farmers, were brilliant.

They kept me informed of their haymaking activities, and for three or four weeks I was prepared to drop everything to document their activities. Fortunately my wife, Chris, knows and loves me. One afternoon we had planned to entertain family to a traditional Sunday lunch for nine of us. At eleven o'clock I was informed by one of my hill-farming friends, "We're

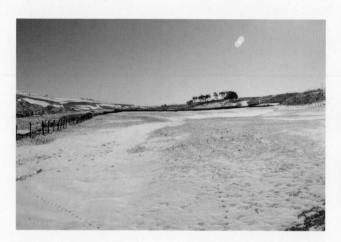

February.

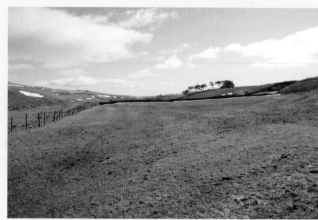

March.

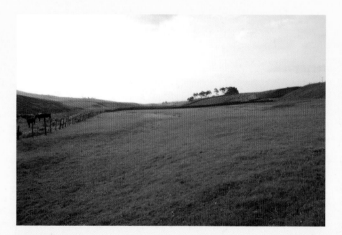

May.

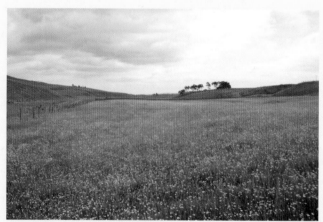

June.

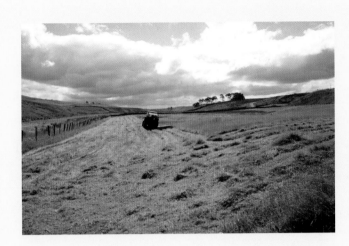

July.

August.

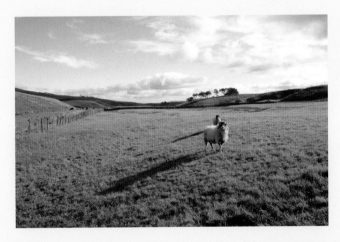

October.

A series of pictures of a traditional hay meadow taken from the same point between February and October.

baling at two o'clock." Chris, without batting an eyelid, served some canapés and postponed lunch till three-thirty pm.

On all of the farms I had chosen to document, the plan was to produce the traditional rectangular bales. Frequent showers rendered this impossible, so my farmers chose instead to bundle the hay/haylage into huge round bales and encase them in plastic wrapping.

This is a wonderful option. For centuries, the hill farmer had to rely on a period of good haymaking weather to ensure the well-being of his stock over the winter. If the weather was not good, poor-quality feed would debilitate the stock. It was a precarious situation every year. Now, for the first time in centuries, the conservation of winter feed is not at the whim of the fickle Pennine weather.

There is a post-script to this tale.

When people talk of "countryside smells", they are usually referring to the rich aroma generated by the spreading of farmyard manure. Some people find it offensive, but I see it as a part of country living. There are many more contributors to the "atmosphere" of country living—new-mown grass, the high-summer memories evoked by a hayshed in winter, the woody drift that hangs in the air after heather-burning.

However, there is one countryside smell that has captivated me since I was a small boy. It's a heady aroma rather like an expensive perfume.

I noticed that it always occurred after a shower of warm spring rain. Eventually I noticed, too, that I always stumbled across it when in a birch wood. But there my detective skills came to an abrupt halt. For years I looked high and low for the source of this captivating assault on my senses. I searched for exotic spring flowers. I crouched down on hands and knees sniffing the turf. The secret of the heady, delicate, slightly musky aroma evaded me for decades.

And then, in an instant, it was solved.

I was reading an article on the flora and vegetation of the dale written by my friend Dr Margaret Bradshaw when I had the Eureka! moment.

I quote Margaret:

❙❙ *A somewhat different birch woodland occurs at Park End. It is of considerable interest to note that some of the birches are of the northern race (Betula pubescens sp*

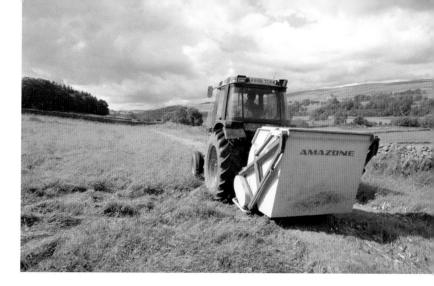

The answer had been under my nose, so to speak, all the time. The heady aroma was not from some elusive botanical inhabitant of the birch wood. It was the birch tree itself that was the source.

Park End Wood is a magical place. Lichen and moss hang from the gnarled branches of the old birches. Huge hazel bushes and delicate rowan punctuate the dominant species. Park End remains as the best example of ancient woodland in the area, much as it was when Neolithic hunter-gatherers came to these hills in about 4000 BC. The heady smell that had haunted me for so long was, indeed, primaeval. It was in the air when man first arrived in the dale.

If you live in northern Britain and have an old birch wood near you, then perhaps it would be worth a visit after a shower of warm spring rain. You might just come across the heady aroma that greeted Stone Age man on his arrival in the Pennines thousands of years ago.

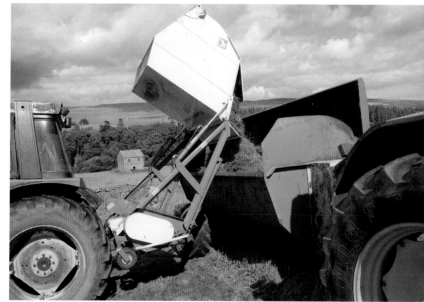

Regeneration of traditional hay meadows. Seeded grass is cut and collected, then transferred to a muck-spreader. It is then taken to a suitable meadow, which has been prepared by scarifying the sward. Cattle are then introduced. Their feet will press the seed heads into the ground.

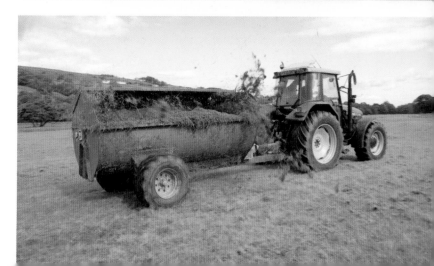

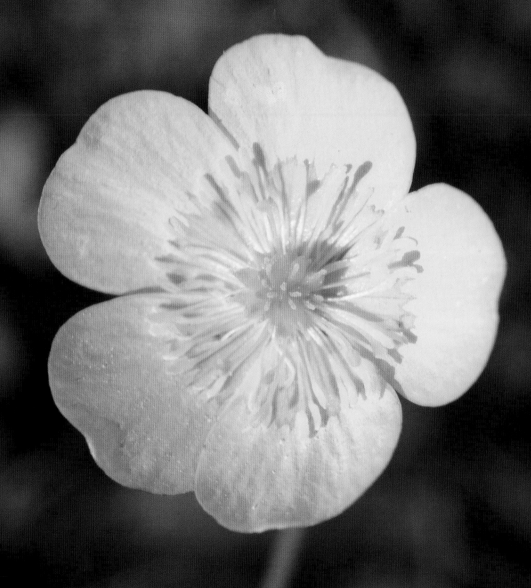

Some hay-meadow flowers.

Meadow buttercup.

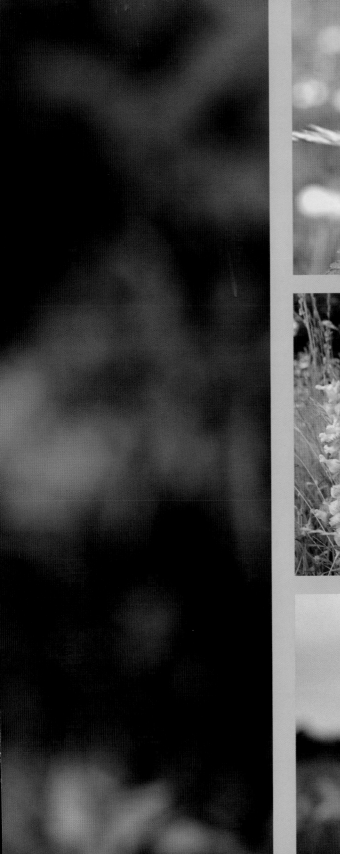

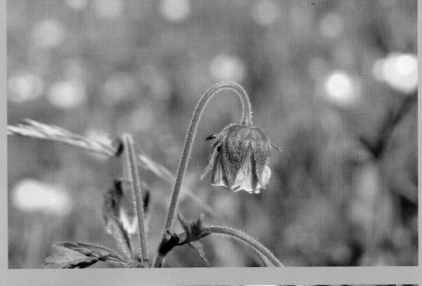

Water avens.

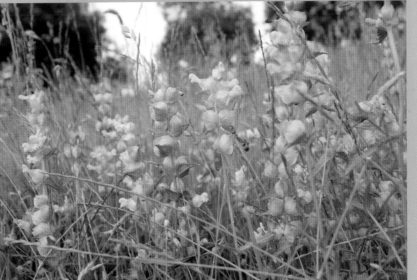

Yellow rattle.

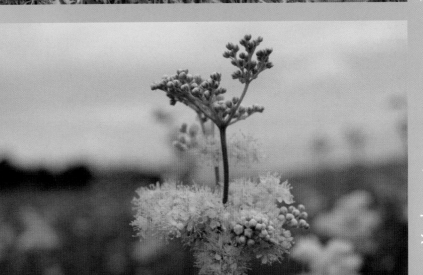

Meadowsweet.

Harebell.

Creeping thistle.

Achillea.

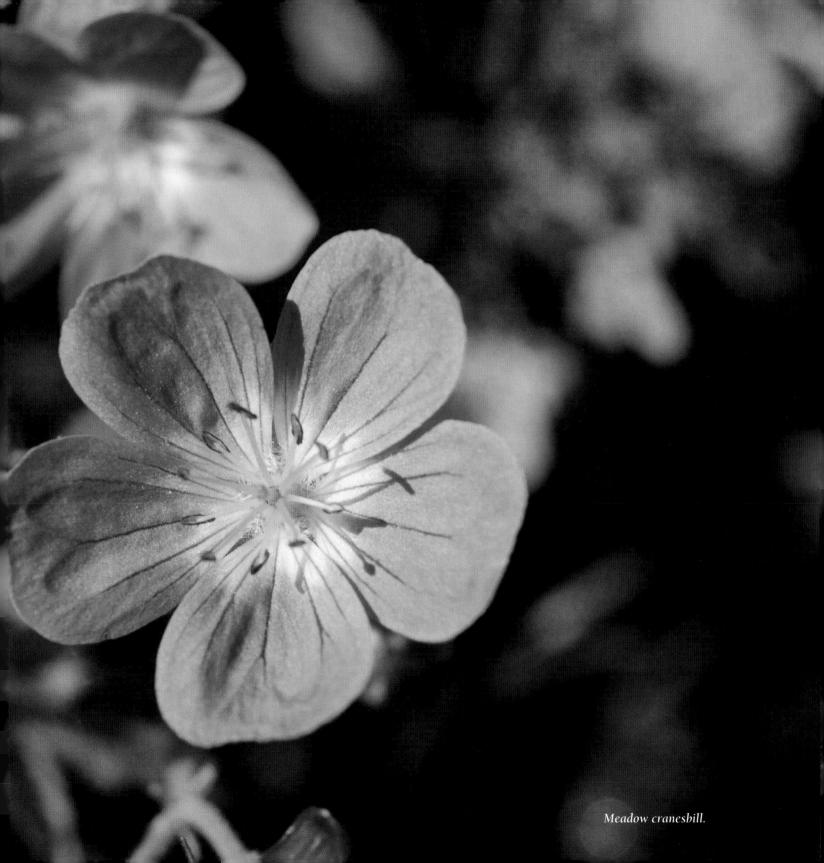

Meadow cranesbill.

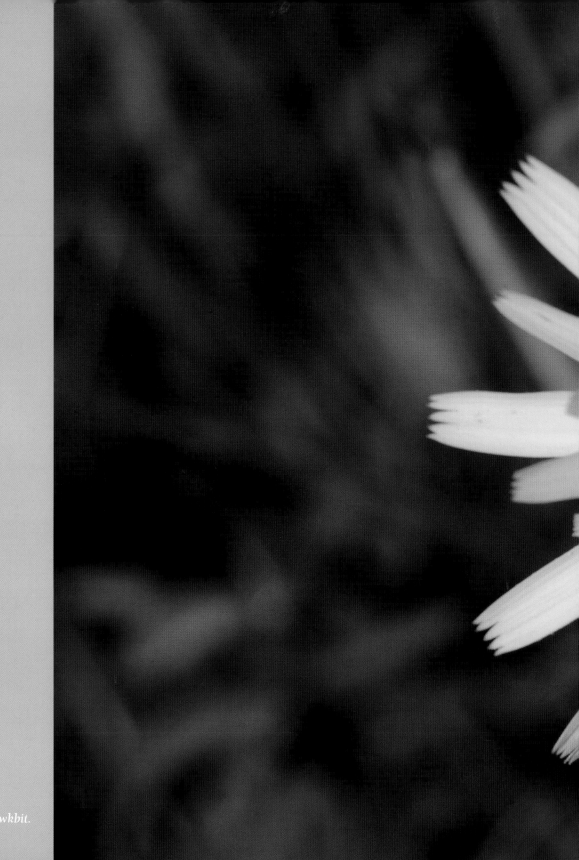

Hawkbit.

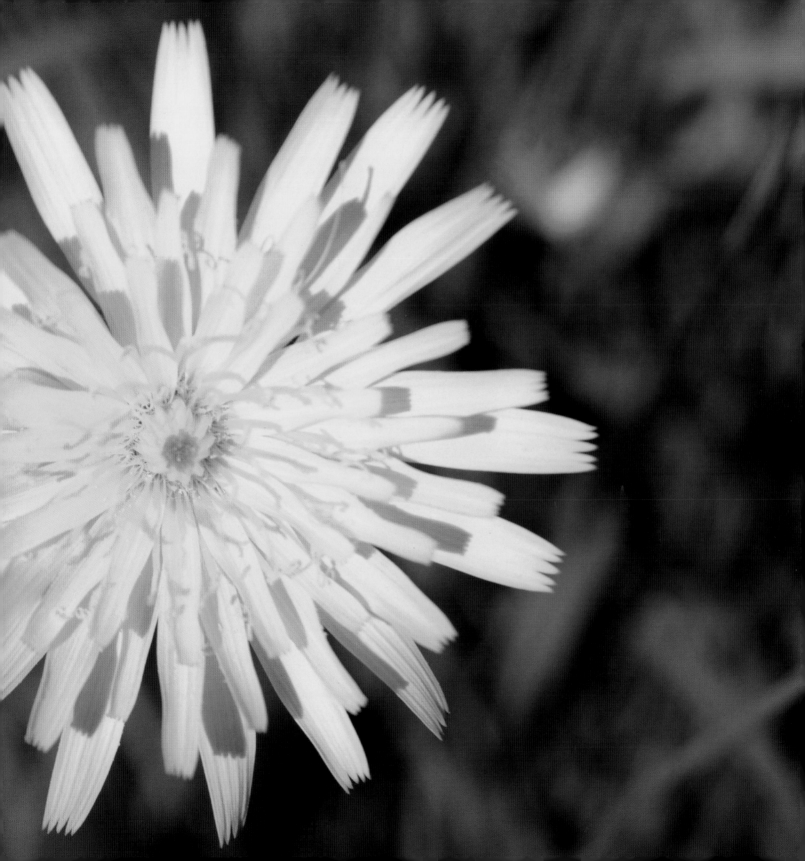

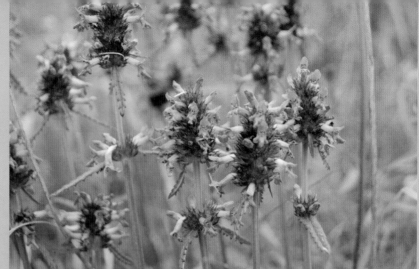

Betony.

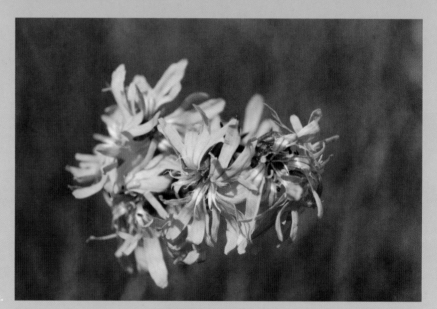

Ragged Robin.

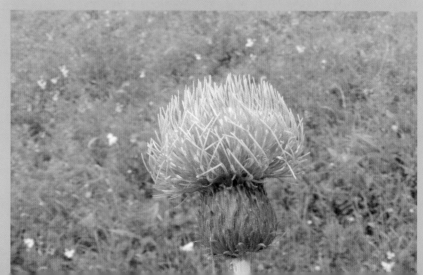

Melancholy thistle.

31 February in the Dale

Drifts of snowdrops, celandines, and aconites in the village churchyard; rooks noisily carrying out repairs to their storm-damaged homes; flocks of wading birds driven by instinct to fly west to their breeding grounds on the hills; toads stirring from their winter dormitories and running the gauntlet across busy roads to reach suitable ponds.

I love the expectancy, the optimism of this time of year. Nature seems to have set deadlines against which appearances must be made, tasks accomplished. There is an urgency for the players to get ahead of the game before spring catches them napping. The rules of the game apply not only to the natural world, but also to the folk who make their living in this countryside. The signs of their activities are, to me, as sure a reminder of the approaching spring as are the snowdrops in the churchyard.

The most obvious of these is heather-burning. When the weather and the wind are right, huge plumes of grey-brown smoke rise from the moors. They seldom occur singly. Sometimes dozens of smoke signals punctuate the horizon, and a fragrant woody tang pervades the whole of the dale as though someone has lit a giant joss stick somewhere.

There is a reason for this urgent flurry of activity. Operations must cease before the ground-nesting birds have started breeding. The burning season runs from October through to the end of March, but

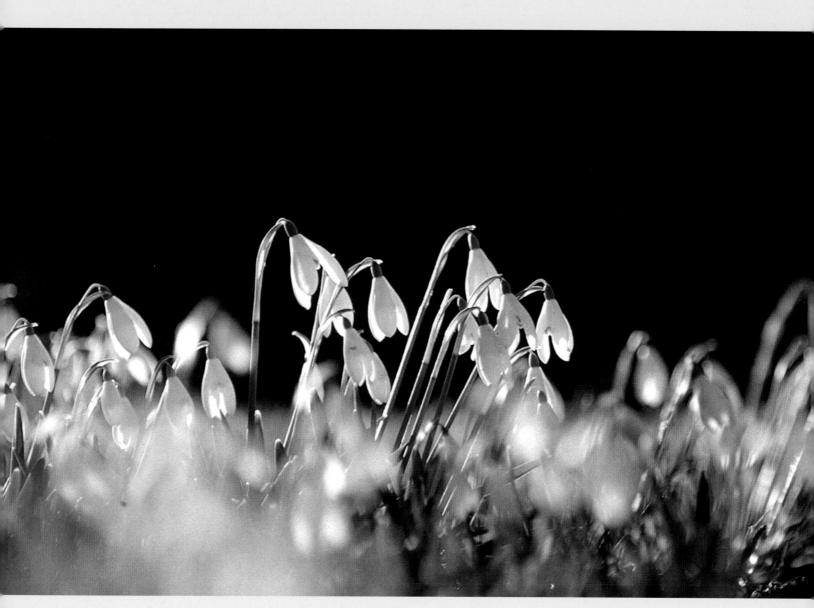

Aconites and snowdrops in a dales churchyard.

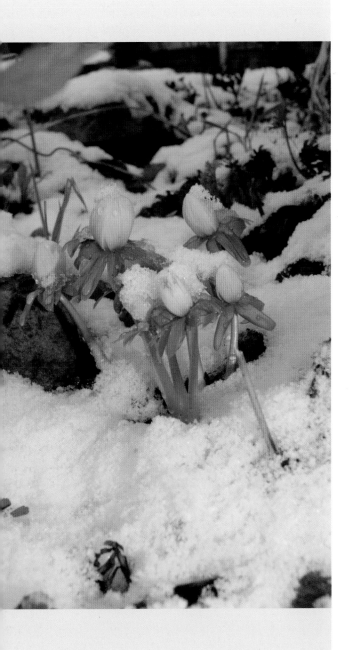

within this period perfect operating conditions are rare. The ground should be wet and the heather dry, with wind of optimum strength. The burn will then remove old woody growth, allowing young nutritious shoots to spring from the rootstock. In addition millions of dormant heather seeds will germinate, stimulated by gentle toasting and exposure to light.

The second frantic human activity at this time of year also adds a distinct tang to the air of the dales, although it could not be described as fragrant or woody. I refer, of course, to "muck-spreading".

Cattle are generally housed for the winter. Whether the housing is in a traditional stone barn or a big modern cowshed, an inevitable mountain of muck accumulates. (In our studies at college it was politely referred to as FYM—farm yard manure.) Its nitrogen-rich content is vital to ensure soil fertility and a good hay crop in the summer. It must be spread on the hay meadows at every opportunity before grass growth begins.

There is a problem in beating nature's deadline. The problem is rain. Dales winters are always wet. The ground becomes saturated. Machinery would destroy the sward.

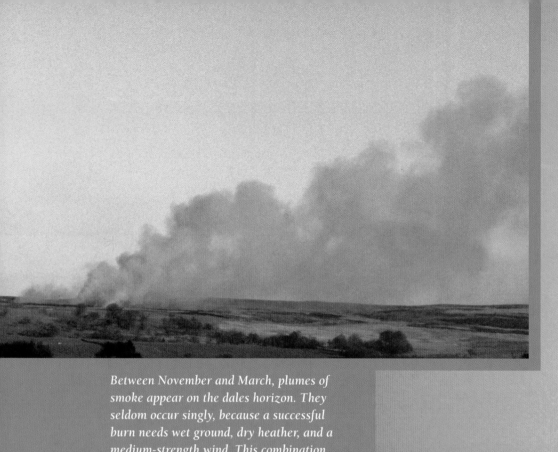

Between November and March, plumes of smoke appear on the dales horizon. They seldom occur singly, because a successful burn needs wet ground, dry heather, and a medium-strength wind. This combination of factors may not occur very often, so the opportunity must be seized.

In *Much Ado About Nothing* Shakespeare sums up February beautifully. "Good morrow, Benedick," says Don Pedro. "Why, what's the matter? That you have such a February face, full of frost, of storm, and cloudiness."

The storm and cloudiness hinder the muck-spreading schedule, but the frost is a bonus. Severe frosts put a rock-hard crust on the fields, allowing access of machinery without damaging the surface.

Until the advent of the tractor, muck-spreading was a long and arduous operation. A low cart would be filled and taken to the meadow, where part of its load would be shed at intervals to leave a field with dozens of piles of manure. A labourer with a gripe would then spread or "scale" each pile so that the manure was fairly evenly distributed. Horse-drawn harrows would then complete the process. Nowadays one man on a tractor can accomplish the task quickly and efficiently.

The third countryman involved in the race against time goes about his task in a much less obvious manner. He is the mole-catcher. His deadline—like that of the muck-spreader—is the spring flush of grass (which will mask his quarry). In a mild winter the fields erupt with mole activity, causing serious problems for the farmer.

Mole-catching is an art. There is an air of mystery about it. As the operator surveys a field blighted by hundreds of molehills, he seems to know instinctively and almost immediately how to lay his traps.

He uses a small spade to cut a square of turf over a tunnel, lays his trap, and replaces the turf. The traps are humane, but also expensive. The mole-catcher will use a "belt and braces" technique to ensure that when he returns in twenty-four hours to check the traps, none is overlooked. He will

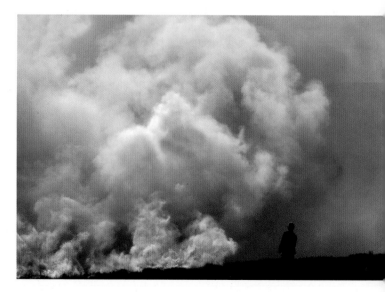

At close quarters the burn can be quite spectacular.

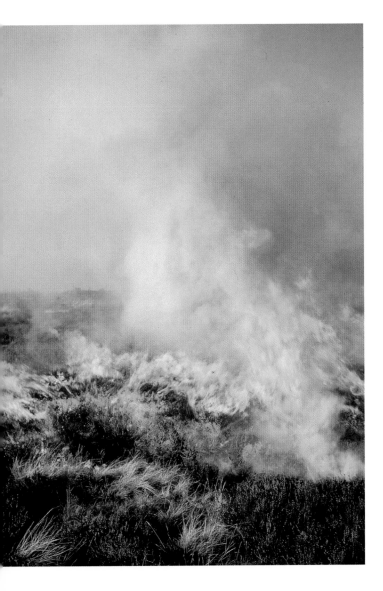

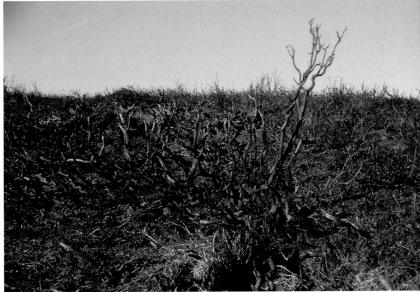

The heat generated can be intense, but the burn soon moves along.

mark each trap with a small flag, but he will also make a sketch map of the whole field, showing where each trap is laid.

And so, while the retreating snowcaps on the hills still bear their signature of winter, the countryside is poised for the arrival of spring. The rooks, the frogs, the curlew, and the countryman are all responding to nature's demands to hit its unrelenting deadlines.

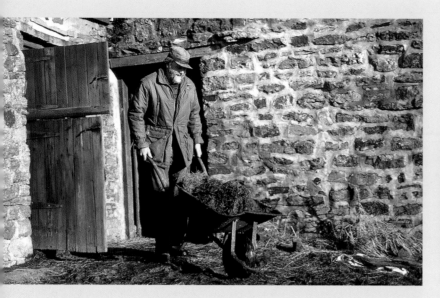

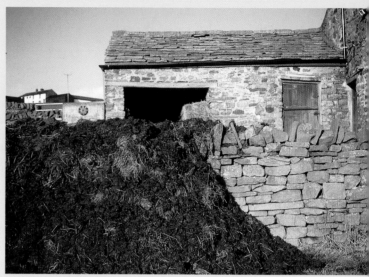

Barrowing manure to the . .   *. . . muckheap.*

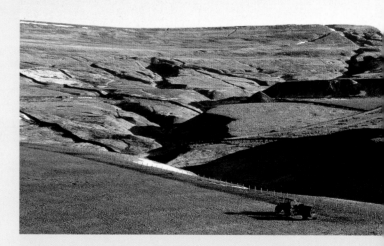

From the muckheap it is transferred to the spreader, which deposits it on the hay meadows.

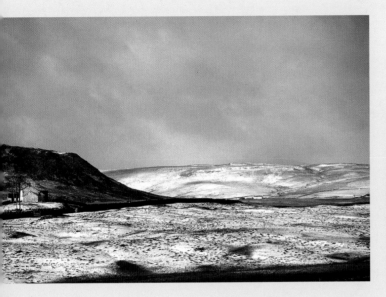

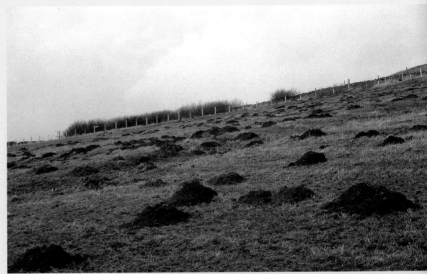

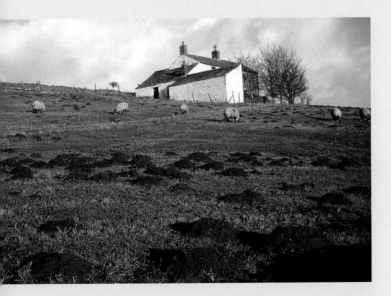

In the early spring the dale erupts with mole activity.

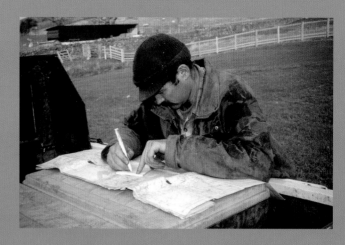

Mapping the position of the traps.

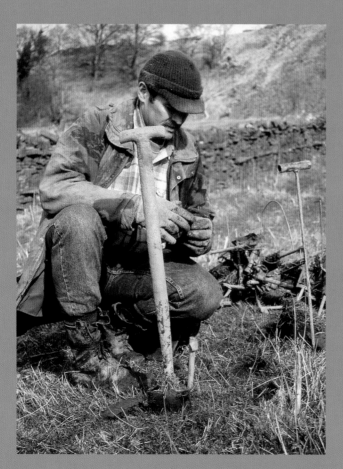

The mole-catcher sets a trap.

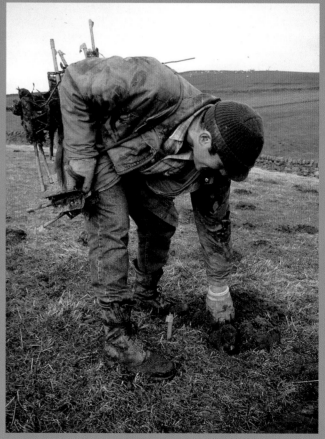

Checking the traps the following morning.

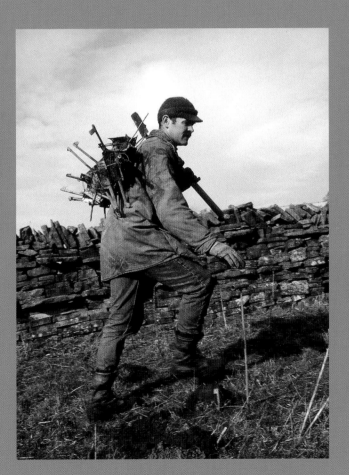

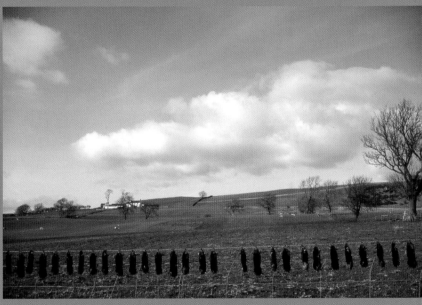

*Traditionally, mole-catchers advertise their skill by leaving
a mole-catcher's gibbet to display their success.*

And so to the next field.

32 Monuments to the Era of the Pack Pony

There remains in the dales a feature of the landscape that is a legacy of the era of the pack pony. It's not quite as obvious as the stone barns that once were used to house stock in the winter. Nor is it as obvious as the thousands of miles of stone walls that stand as a reminder of the enclosure acts.

Between October and April, for six months of the year, many of the dales roads were a quagmire, making wheeled transport impossible, so the only feasible method of carrying goods was by pack pony. Since the dales were criss-crossed by hundreds of rivers and streams (termed "becks"), there are hundreds of pack-horse bridges on the old pack-horse routes. These sturdy stone structures with elegant arches tend to be tucked away, hidden in steep-sided valleys (termed "gills").

Some of these bridges date back to mediaeval times. They are very easily identified. Never more than six feet wide (a dimension that would preclude wheeled traffic), they have very low parapets so as not to interfere with the bulky packs on each side of the pony. Their structure is a work of art.

Strings of up to twenty ponies would transport goods throughout the dale. They were very important in the lead industry, which flourished for the whole of the nineteenth century. Ore would be carried to the smelter, and then lead ingots would be transferred to water transport. On the return journey their panniers would be loaded with fuel for the furnace.

These bridges remain as a dales monument to the hundreds of years when "horsepower" really meant horsepower.

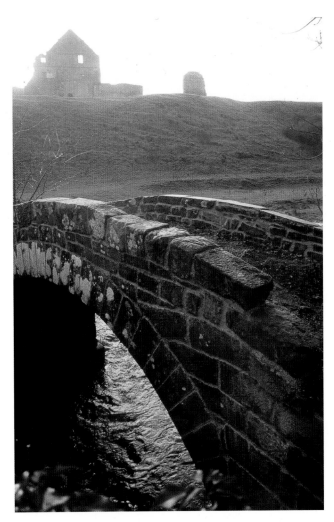

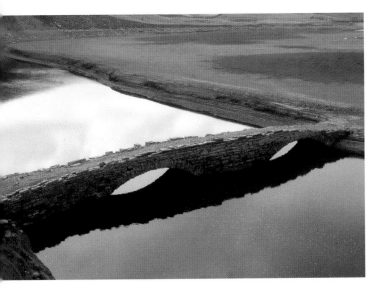

This is an unusual pack-horse bridge in that it has two arches.

The pack-horse bridge below Eggleston Abbey. It spans the Thorsgill Beck.

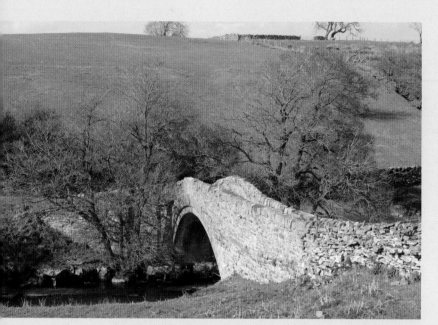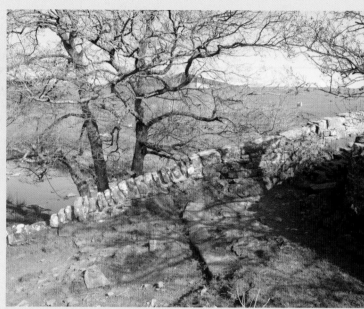

These pictures of the bridge over Deepdale Beck demonstrate the three characteristics of pack-horse bridges: an elegant arch, a narrow roadway, and low parapets.

33 On the Rocks

The role of geology in the making of a unique dale

My love of the Teesdale landscape deepened over the years. Every journey west from the practice base at Barnard Castle increased my sense of awe at what is truly a unique landscape. I marvelled at how the dale had reached this pinnacle of beauty over a vast time-scale, and anxiously read all I could on the subject.

It's hard to imagine that 350 million years ago the Pennine hills were on the Equator.

For 50 million years our landscape spent much of the time under a warm tropical sea full of primaeval invertebrates. As these organisms died, their calcium-rich skeletons accumulated on the sea bed in deep layers which have today become limestone. Conditions were constantly changing, and the warm tropical sea gave way to shallow estuaries where aggregations of granular sediment washed down. Over millions of years this became sandstone. If the sediment was muddy, this was transformed into shale. And where lush, swampy forest developed, this became the coal layers that give their name to that geological era, the carboniferous period.

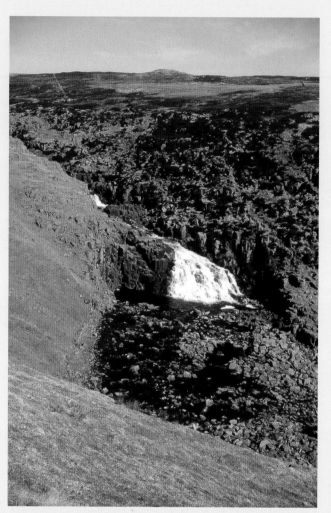

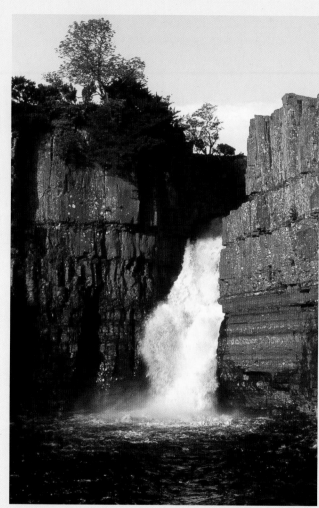

The infant Tees flows down a channel in the basalt at Cauldron Snout.

At High Force the basalt can be seen overlying limestone strata.

These alternations happened over and over many times, so that there are repeated series of these four types of carboniferous rock.

And then, at the end of the carboniferous period, about 295 million years ago, there was violent movement of the earth's tectonic plates resulting in huge amounts of volcanic activity. Molten rock at over a thousand degrees was pushed up through cracks in the carboniferous strata. In spite of enormous pressure it did not reach the surface, but was squeezed between the limestone layers where it solidified into hard basalt. Gradually the softer limestone and sandstone eroded to leave huge slabs of volcanic rock, up to eighty metres thick, exposed in the landscape.

The intrusion of hard volcanic dolerite, known as the Great Whin Sill, occurs in a diagonal line across north-east England, taking in Teesdale, Weardale, Hadrian's Wall, and the Farne Islands. In places, where the molten basalt came into contact with limestone, the heat transformed the limestone into a granular form known as sugar limestone.

This sugar limestone underlies much of the thin soil of Upper Teesdale and is a major factor in the unique assortment of plant species that flourish

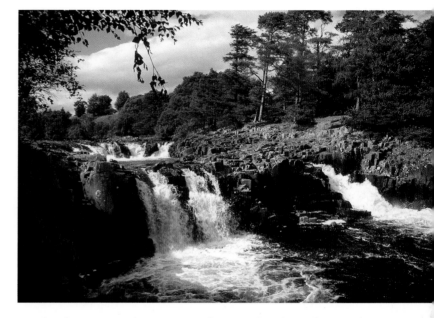

Further downstream the river cascades over the whin sill.

there. The hard, impervious whinstone covered by shallow soil prevented the growth of trees, so that in the post-glacial landscape the alpine flora survived in this very special isolated ecosystem. Elsewhere in Britain, as scrub and forest developed, the alpine plants were overgrown and disappeared from the landscape.

Nurtured by its physical surroundings and a cool microclimate of its own, the upper dale has become internationally renowned by botanists who

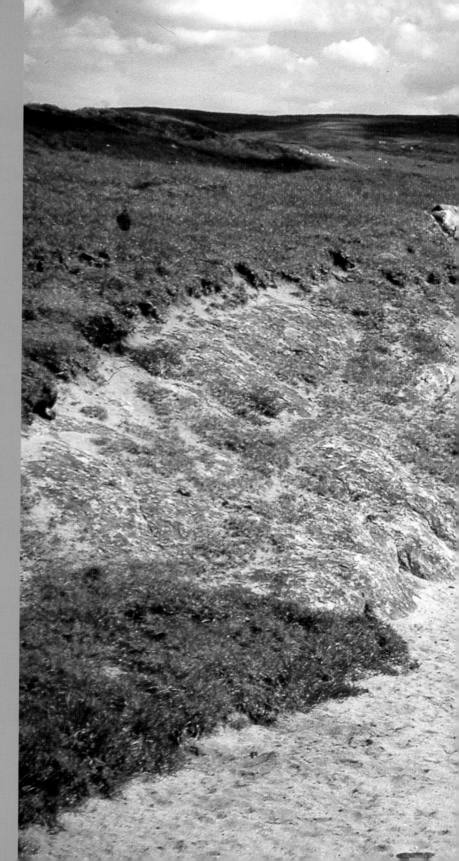

Where the molten rock contacted limestone, the heat converted the limestone into a granular form called "sugar limestone". This underlies much of the upper dale, and is a factor in the "Teesdale Assemblage", a unique population of botanical species including many alpine plants.

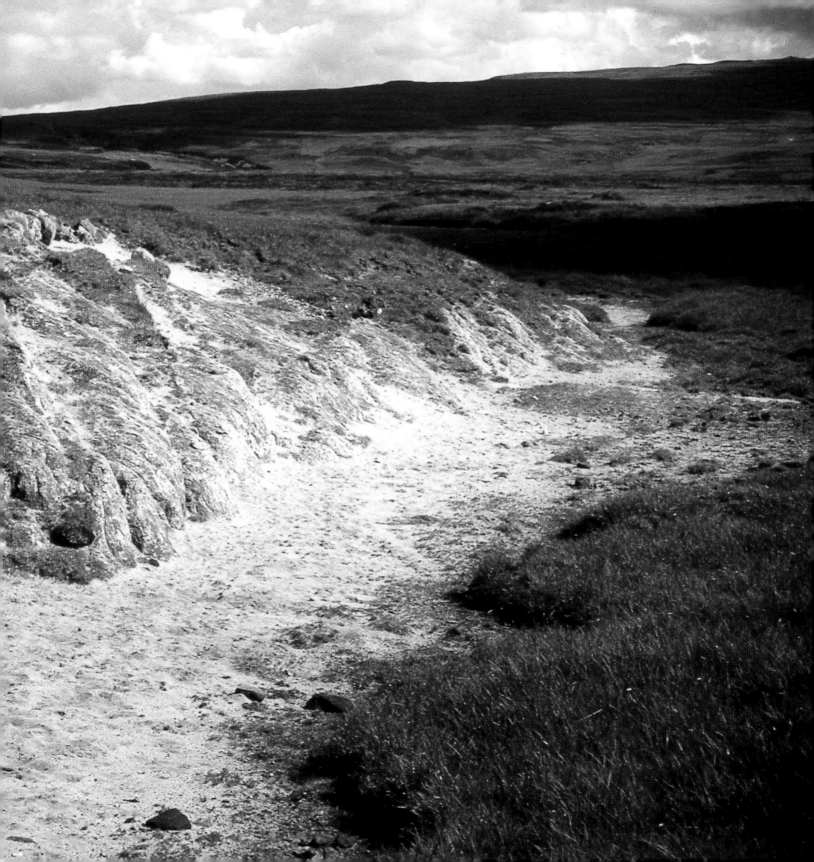

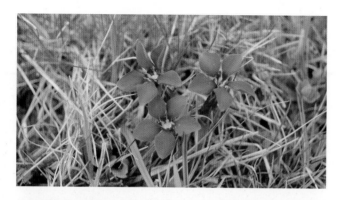

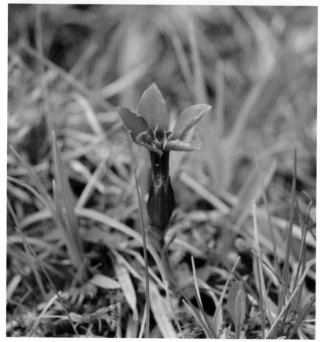

The spring gentian (Gentiana verna), which appears in May. To many it is the emblem of Teesdale.

come from all over the world to see the "Teesdale Assemblage".

The star of the show, and an emblem of Teesdale, is the blue gentian. Whilst it is common in mountainous areas like the Jura, the Balkans, and the High Atlas of Morocco, it is rare in Britain, being found only in Teesdale and a few locations in the west of Ireland. It is a tiny plant, about five centimetres tall, with a beautiful vivid blue flower appearing in May.

The list of rare plants is extensive, and includes thrift, hoary rock rose, mountain avens, dwarf birch, Jacob's ladder, sea plantain, cloudberry, yellow mountain saxifrage, Scottish asphodel, bird's-eye primrose and spring sandwort. Many give a clue to their origins with names such as alpine bartsia, alpine foxtail, alpine bistort, and alpine meadow-rue.

Because of their isolation, some of the plants have evolved into distinct varieties. The hairs on the foliage of the hoary rock rose are of a different type and distribution to its relatives outside of the dale. The shrubby cinquefoil has its Teesdale variant. Even the spring gentian has its own local peculiarities. Of the nine species of alchemilla

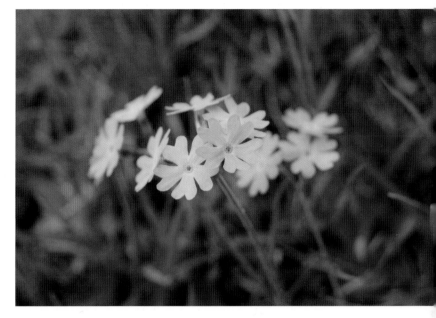

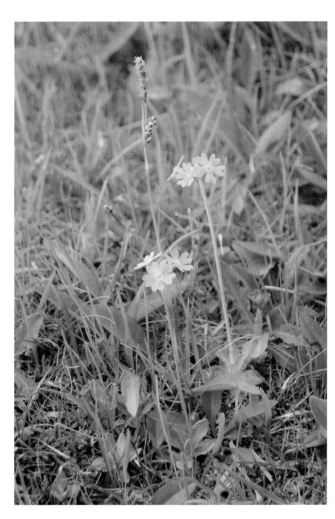

The bird's-eye primrose (Primula farinosea).

found in the Assemblage, two are unique to Teesdale. A species of violet, Viola rupestris, is known worldwide as the Teesdale violet.

In 1961, as an A-level botany student, I was taken on a field trip to an area in the upper dale known as Cow Green to see the wonderful Teesdale Assemblage. Even then it was suspected that this area was under threat and could end up under millions of gallons of water. On 8 December 1964 the Tees Valley and Cleveland Water Board announced formally that their new reservoir would be built at Cow Green. Conservationists launched the "Battle for Cow Green", but it was to no avail.

Preliminary work started in 1967, and by 1971 the reservoir was filled. Seven hundred and seventy acres of land, stretching for two miles, disappeared under 9,000 million gallons of water. Twenty-one of those acres were home to some very rare plants. The work of the conservationists, although failing to halt development of the reservoir, did much to raise the profile of Upper Teesdale's importance and since then the remaining landscape has gained strict environmental protection.

Apart from the whin sill's part in creating a botanist's delight, it has given rise to some striking features in the dale's landscape, particularly the waterfalls of the Tees.

Just below Cow Green reservoir is "Cauldron Snout", Britain's highest cataract, where the river tumbles two hundred feet over angular basalt.

Adjacent to it is a seventy-metre-high slab of whinstone known as "Falcon Clints". Further downstream is High Force, one of Britain's most spectacular waterfalls, where the juxtaposition of the whin sill and the carboniferous layers can be clearly seen. And yet further downstream is Low Force, a bubbling, surging series of cascades over the dark volcanic rocks.

All the Pennine dales are beautiful. All are different. All have spectacular features in their landscape. Before the invention of the internal combustion engine, each was a crucible in which style, culture, and architecture evolved separately from that of neighbouring dales.

Perhaps I'm biased, but Teesdale is the dale closest to my heart. I regard it as special. And there are many geologists and botanists who would certainly agree with me.

34 Into the Light

Sunset and Sunrise in the Dales

I remember well the very first picture of a sunrise that I ever took. It was in June 1960. I know the date because I was up very early, sitting on a stool at the front door of my home, swotting for my O-levels.

In the minutes before the sun appeared, the sky's colours and the haze of a midsummer morning made a breath-taking scene. Even in those days my camera was never far away, and I caught the view with my Kodak Colorsnap as the sun breached the horizon. Despite such basic equipment, the results were quite good. The glorious colours of the morning had been captured. However, as a pleasing, well-composed picture it was seriously lacking. The flat roof of a modern sports pavilion and a few treetops in the foreground had done nothing to enhance a moment of wonderful natural beauty.

It was a lesson learned, rewarded many times by stimulating an eye for the prospect of a good sunrise or sunset, and searching for an interesting silhouette in the foreground to complete a pleasing composition.

The classic conditions occur after a warm summer's day when, as the day draws to a close, a mist or haze forms on the horizon. With luck there will follow twenty to thirty minutes of pure magic as

I love taking pictures of sunsets, but it's a real challenge to be in the right place at the right time to frame a good picture. Catching a dramatic landscape composition often happens by chance. I particularly like the one that looks as though the sun is a big golden ball rolling down a hill.

Another favourite
foreground interest
is trees. They can be
sculptural or skeletal.
I'm particularly fond of
the one where the sun is
shining through a dense
mist giving a monochrome
picture through the limbs
of a dead tree.

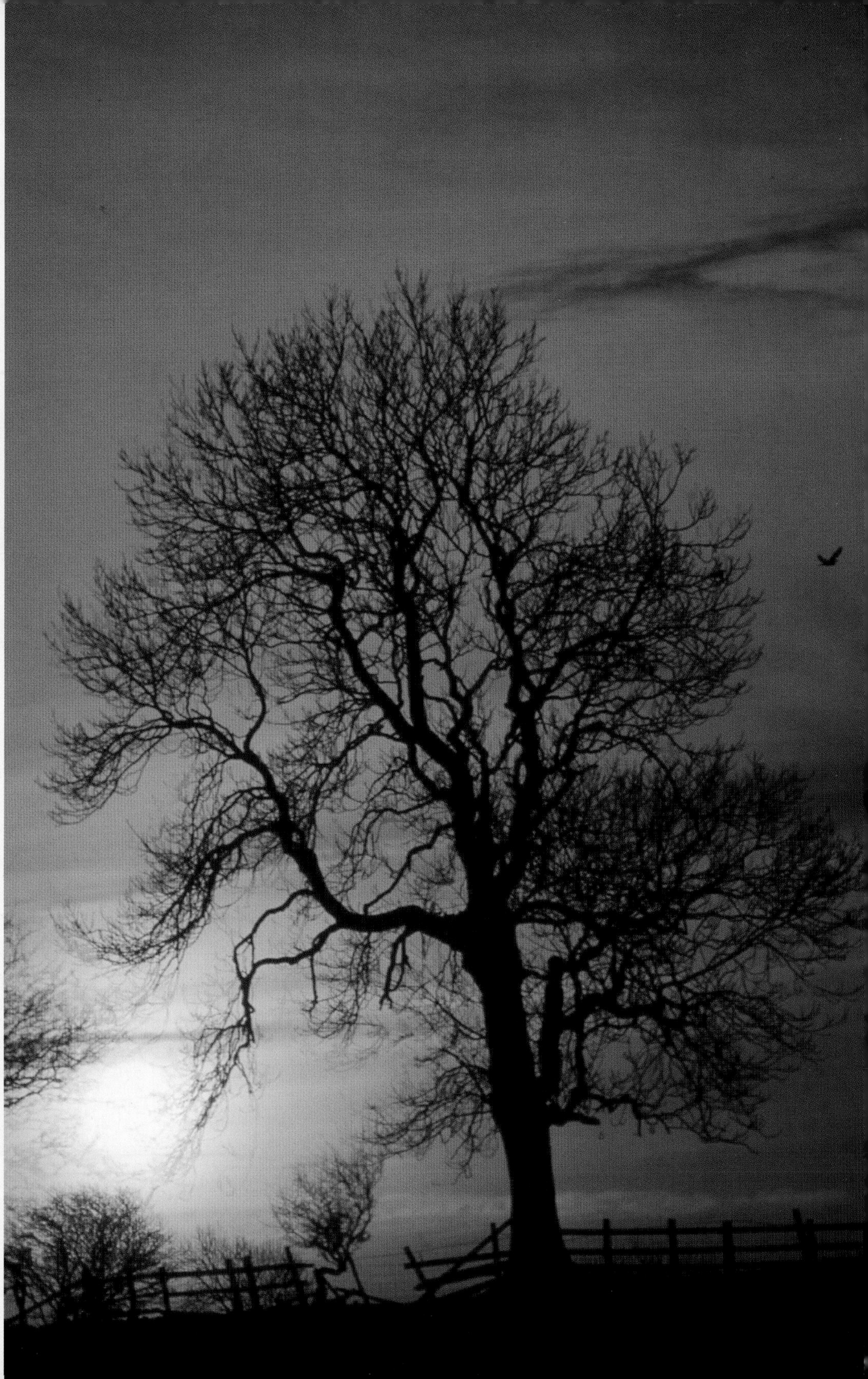

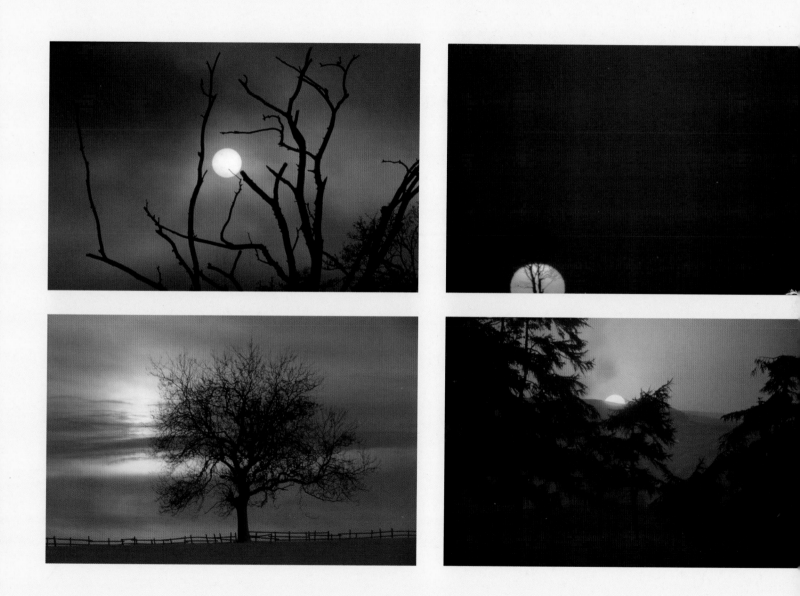

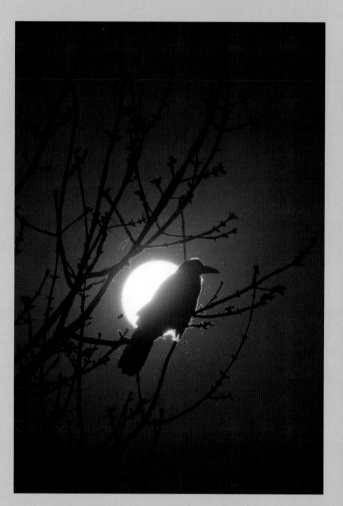

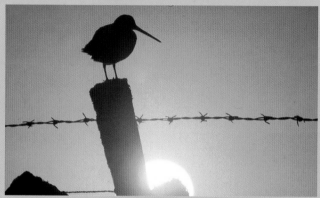

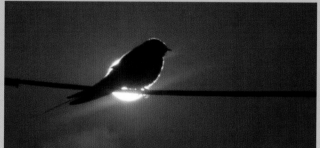

*Landscapes and trees stand still but birds tend to fly away
as I approach, presenting something of a challenge. Here
we see a snipe on a fencepost, a rook in a tree, a swallow
on a wire, a meadow pipit hopping along a stone wall, and
a curlew in majestic pose.*

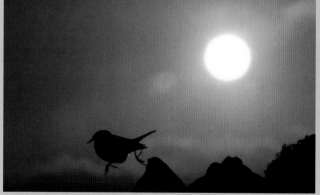

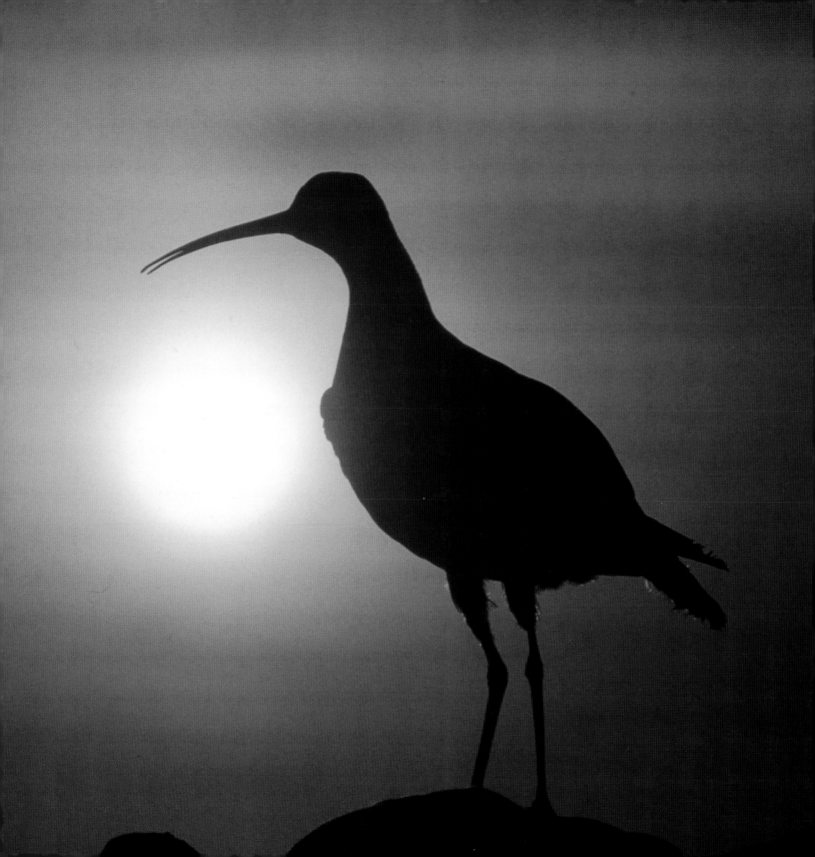

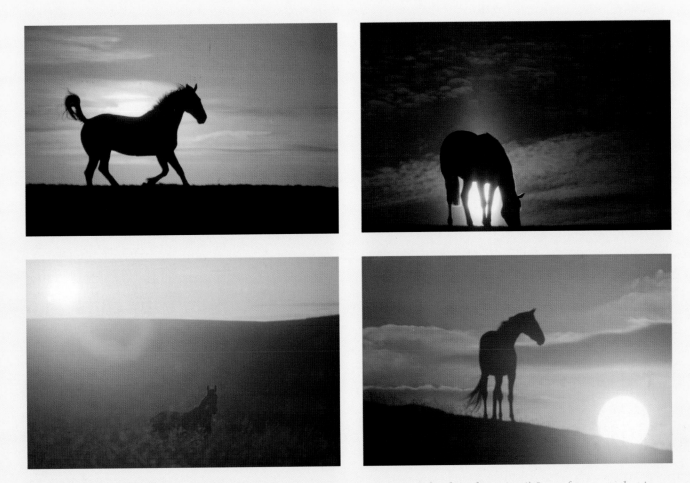

The ultimate iconic silhouette is the horse. (There's a bank that has known this for a long time!) I was fortunate that in my travels in the dales I could make a mental note of possibilities, and follow them up. The last one in this sequence is the one that took weeks of observation, but did win a national photographic competition.

the sun dips into this ethereal haze, and turns itself into a fiery, glowing orb.

Guessing the flight path of this orb, monitoring its dimming intensity, and getting into the right place at the right time is a great game, and Teesdale is a wonderful place to play this game. Being on the east of the Pennines, the sun throws its diminishing light from the west over serried ranks of hills, with the dales landscape in the foreground. There are so many features that can be included: the natural contours of the hills, old fieldhouses, village churches, trees, a landscape peppered with livestock. The list is endless.

Introducing animals or birds into the composition adds a whole new dimension to the game. It requires quick thinking, and a camera in the hand, ready to shoot. Perhaps a curlew will paraglide across the sky, or a short-eared owl will quarter the moor.

My absolute favourite shot was taken at sunrise on a midsummer morning.

Many years ago I was impressed by a handsome horse in a field near the village of Eggleston. There was a knoll in the middle of the field, and I imagined the horse striking a pose on this knoll with a rising sun behind it. For a period of weeks I took an avid interest in the weather forecast, and if conditions looked promising I would set my internal alarm clock to survey the pre-dawn sky. If all was well I would travel to the spot to be in the right position just before sunrise. Often there would be a superb sunrise but no horse! At other times the horse would stroll onto the knoll as the sun disappeared behind a bank of cloud.

Eventually everything fell into place. One morning the sun rose majestically through the dawn haze, and just as it did so, my subject appeared at just the right spot.

The excitement was such that I had difficulty holding the camera steady. I threw myself down and wedged my elbows into the turf to form a sort of tripod. I had about two minutes of frantic snapping before the horse moved on and the sun emerged from the haze to assume an unfriendly glare.

The results were terrific; well worth the effort. And one of the pictures won a national photographic competition!

35 The Agricultural Show

As summer in the Pennines rolls towards autumn, there begins a succession of agricultural shows.

Almost every weekend, members of the practice give up their free time to do the "Hon Vet" duties, and perhaps some judging.

I loved my days at the show: meeting old friends; catching up with the news; proud to be a part of a special community.

Everyone breathes a sigh of relief when show day dawns dry and bright. A whole year's organisation has gone into setting up this event. A sunny day will assure financial success, with huge gate receipts and loyal support from almost everyone in the dale. However, the hard-working show committee have taken steps to avoid a weather-disaster. Whist drives, domino drives, dinners, and dinner dances have been held to swell the funds, providing a safety net against a wet and windy show day with only a few brave souls in attendance.

I used to take my "Hon Vet" duties very seriously. I'd call at the surgery very early to pick up all the drugs and dressings that I might need for any emergency, and I'd be on the show field as the first horse boxes and cattle trailers appeared. Loading and unloading animals can precipitate accidents.

My first port of call was the secretary's caravan. "Hon Vet reporting for duty," I'd announce.

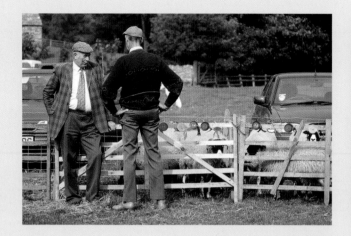

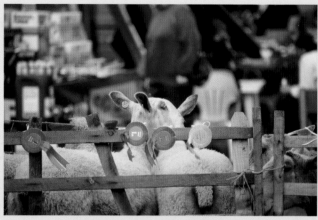

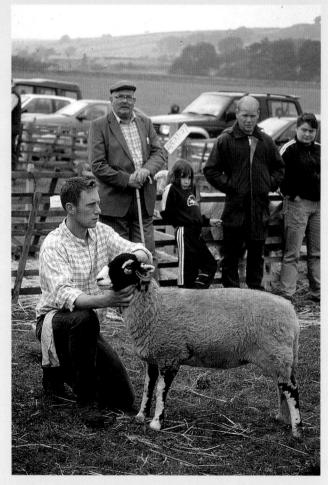

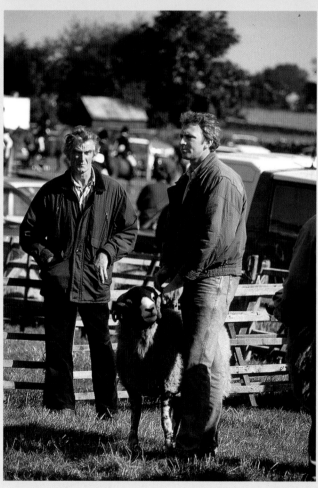

The sheep classes are a serious affair.

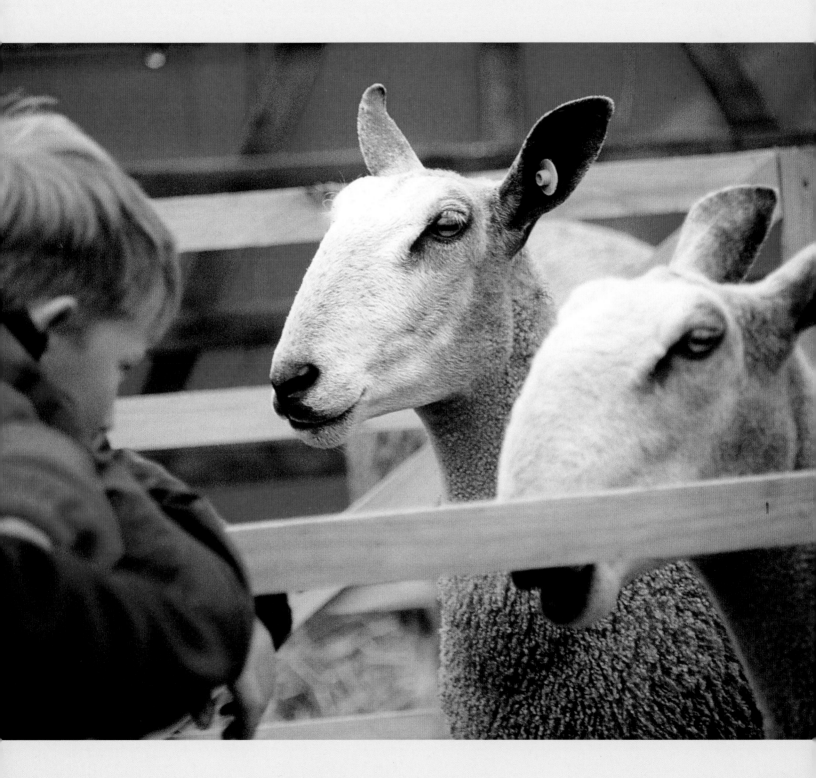

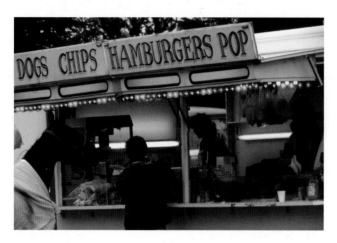

A stop for refreshment. The horse looks as though he'd like a drink, too.

The secretary would provide me with my official badge, a programme, and tickets for lunch and tea. After that I was free to circulate, meeting up with friends I hadn't seen since last show day, watching the judging, and soaking up the atmosphere. All the while I had one ear cocked to the PA system for the echoing words, "Will the veterinary surgeon please report to the . . ."

Thankfully incidents were few and far between, although I vividly remember a greyhound which was suffering from heatstroke, having been shut in a car on a hot day. The poor dog was in convulsions which at any moment could have proved terminal. I administered appropriate drugs, but what saved its life was a water trough I spotted a hundred yards away. With a little help we carried the patient to the trough and plunged his whole body in the icy water. The results were spectacular, with the dog recovering his senses in minutes.

The marquees housing the Industrial section, Horticultural section, and Fur and Feather section opened to the public at midday, the judging having been completed. It would take an hour or two to do them justice, noting in particular friends who have won prizes.

As the last horsebox left the field I could at last relax, and bask in the memories of another convivial show day.

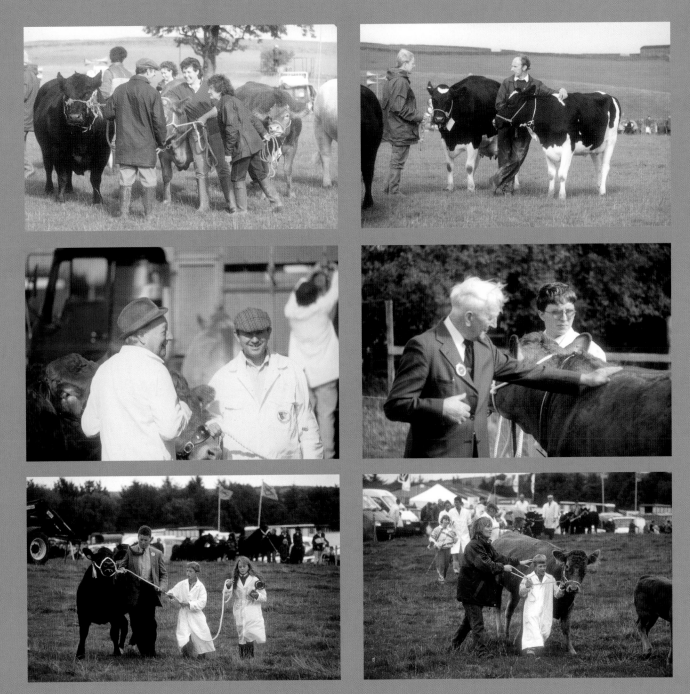

The cattle classes have a much more relaxed atmosphere.

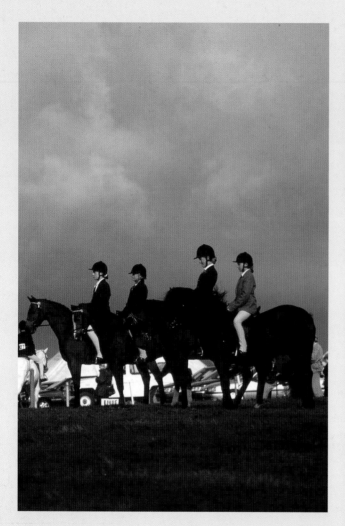

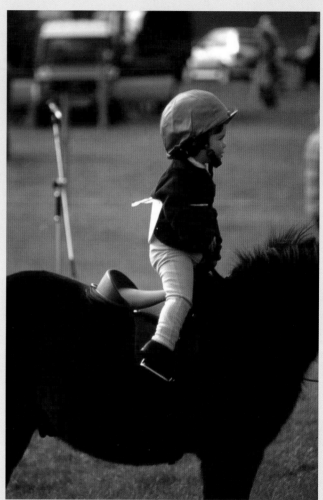

The pony classes attract young and old alike.

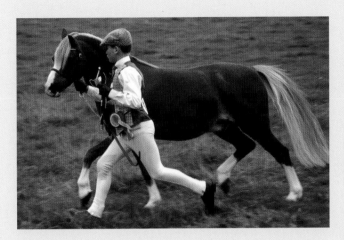

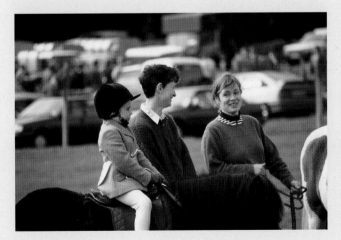

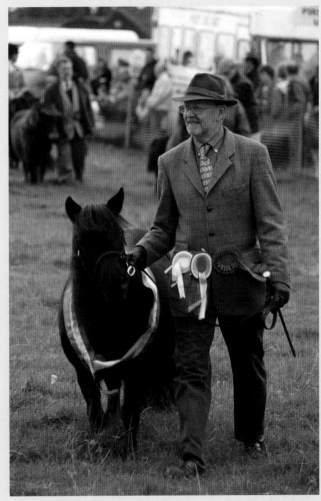

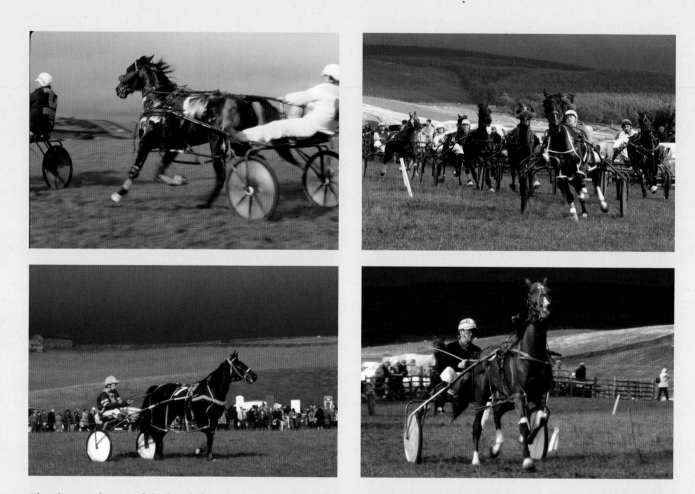

The climax of some of the local shows is grass-track trotting races. Brave drivers hurtle round the uneven track on the flimsiest of rigs, which seem little more than a tractor seat and a pair of bicycle wheels.

It's rather like the chariot race in Ben-Hur.

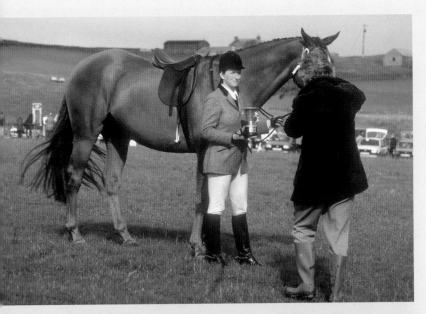

Since 1854 the Teesdale Mercury *has published the weekly digest of everything that's going on in the dale. Thirty years ago the iconic multitasking editor, chief photographer and chief reporter was Jim McTaggart, and on show day he was everywhere. The results of every section would be faithfully recorded and published the following Wednesday.*

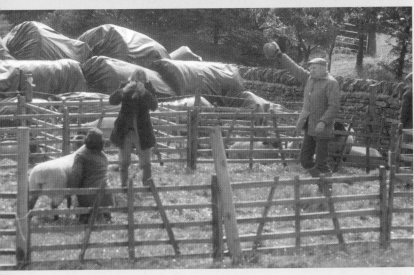

36 Diversification— A Key to Survival

Many years ago my elder son came home from school protesting strongly that he had been unjustly punished for a minor misdemeanour in class. I listened sympathetically to Arthur's account, and it was fairly clear that the guilty party had emerged from the incident scot free, while Arthur had taken the rap. The incident and punishment had been so minor that no further action was necessary.

"But it's not fair," my son protested.

I agreed and groped for some sympathetic and fatherly advice.

"Sometimes life isn't fair," was the best I could muster.

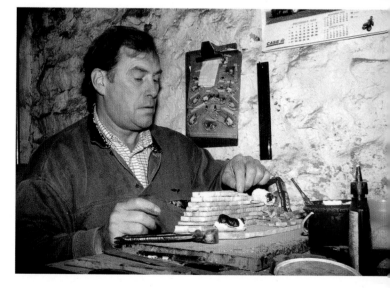

Trevor has turned a hobby into a successful business. Because he is a farmer and an accomplished stone-waller, his models look like the real thing.

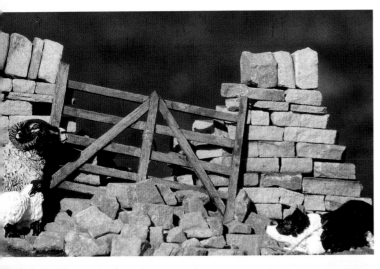

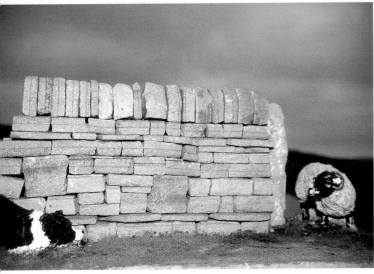

I am reminded of my punchline all those years ago when I reflect on the difficulties that have beset farming in recent years. Most of these difficulties have been inflicted, like my son's punishment, on an innocent party.

I have a great affection for the hill farmer, and admire his hard work and resilience, although these qualities have been sorely tested by global events far from the Pennine hills.

Who would have thought that the fall of the Berlin Wall would send ripples across the North Sea to be felt in the upper reaches of the Pennine Dales years later? But it did. The events in Berlin heralded the disintegration of the USSR and the collapse of the Russian economy. Overnight a market for millions of sheepskins disappeared.

Currency fluctuations had devastating effects on export markets, whilst directives from Brussels and bureaucracy from Westminster have made life increasingly difficult for the farmer.

I suppose the real body blow was BSE. In spite of speculation, no one really knows exactly how or why it happened. But again it had nothing to do with the farmer.

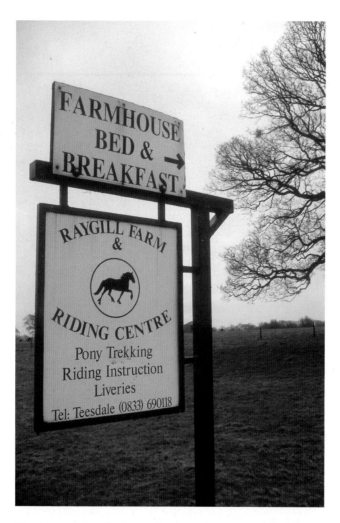

Tourist accommodation and equestrian centre rolled into one.

However, this is not a review of negative or depressing circumstances. It's a celebration of the qualities of resilience and hard work in the face of adversity. My friend the hill farmer hasn't just sat back and moaned about his plight. He's stirred himself and done something about it.

Wives may have taken a job to alleviate cash flow. Some have resurrected professional qualifications in nursing or teaching. Others have skills in dressmaking, catering, and sugarcraft. The farmer himself may have taken part-time employment while still running the farm. However, for many, the key to survival has been diversification. In an already busy life, a further business venture has been developed to shore up diminishing returns from farming. The ingenuity, talent, and energy that have emerged has been amazing.

This was not a new situation for the dales farmer. In the previous century meagre income from the farm was shored up by additional cash flow. Then it was lead-mining and stone-walling. Today the diversification is much more imaginative.

At least two clients capitalised on their skill with a camera.

Colin has a great love and knowledge of the dales landscape and has a flair for capturing its moods on film. He markets his pictures as framed prints, postcards, and attractive tablemats through a shop run by a craft co-operative.

John uses his photographic talents in other directions. As well as being widely published in the farming press with his pictures of prizewinners at shows and markets, he became one of the most accomplished wedding photographers in the area. While John handles the technical side, his wife, Gillian, handles the "people-management", assembling the right people into the right place for the formal portraits. They're quite a team and the results are excellent.

Some have opted for direct marketing of their produce.

Brian is a trained butcher, and opened a butcher's shop on his farm to sell home-reared produce. However, Brian's entrepreneurial flair doesn't stop there. He has converted a disused barn into a bunkhouse where hikers travelling the Pennine Way can stop overnight. The facilities are basic but ideal for the backpacker needing just somewhere to cook, shower, and lay out a sleeping bag. Alongside

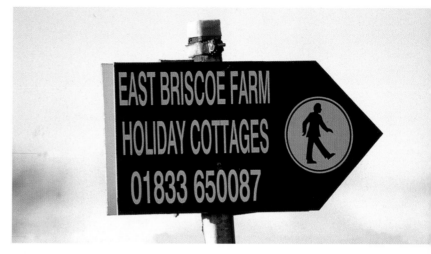

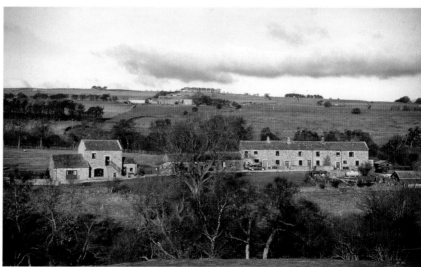

Many redundant farm buildings in the dales have been converted to attractive holiday cottages.

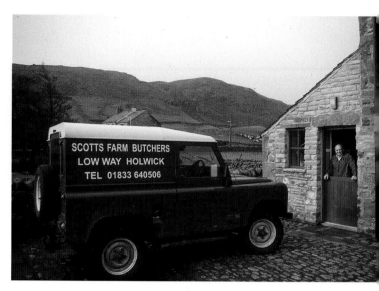

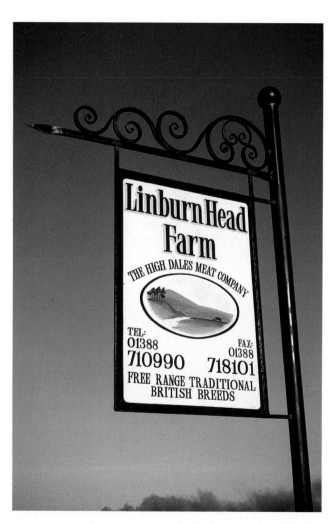

Direct marketing is another successful example of diversification.

the barn he has also created a campsite. As an additional enterprise he has even converted one of his farm buildings into a successful restaurant.

The restaurant is only one of many farm buildings converted to serve the tourist trade. Plenty of barns have been transformed into attractive holiday cottages serving the increase in visitors to the dale. One of the most impressive is in a pretty village where a complex of cowsheds and stables has become a seven-bedroom/five-bathroom luxury cottage.

Trevor, like many hillfarmers, has spent a lot of time building and repairing dry-stone walls. In recent years he has adapted his walling skills to reproduce these structures in miniature. Each piece is unique, and captures cleverly the flavour of the dales landscape. As Dalestone Crafts developed, Trevor incorporated scale-model sheep, lambs, and collies into his creations to make them even more attractive and authentic.

Graeme's story is perhaps the most impressive. His enterprise was so successful that he eventually gave up farming to concentrate on his new business.

Years ago, whilst on a family holiday in the Scottish Highlands, Graeme spent a half day on an off-road driving course. He thoroughly enjoyed the experience and couldn't help noting that while twenty acres of his ninety-acre farm were totally unsuitable for dairy farming, they would make an ideal off-road training ground.

It was just a germ of an idea, and he had neither the time nor the inclination to develop it. He was happy in his work and immensely proud of his fifty-strong herd of top-quality, high-yielding pure-bred Holstein cows. The long hours and the routine of milking twice a day for 365 days a year were accepted as part of the job. It was a way of life, it provided a great deal of job satisfaction, and as long as there was a living in it, Graeme was a happy man.

But the 1990s were nightmare years for all farmers. Every branch of agriculture was assailed by crisis. Incomes from all sectors plummeted.

The frightening scenario unfolded where, in many cases, no matter how hard the farmer worked, there was no longer a viable income to be gained from his agricultural enterprise.

Eventually Graeme realised that the income from dairy farming alone had reached a point where it was no longer sufficient to support his family. Remembering his off-road experience in Scotland, he investigated the development of his twenty acres of rough land into an off-road driving school.

Determined to do the job properly, he signed up for the official off-road driving course run by Land Rover at their Solihull base. It is jokingly referred to as the "Jungle Experience" and incorporates some really difficult conditions. Later he took part in their advanced course at Eastnor in the Malvern Hills.

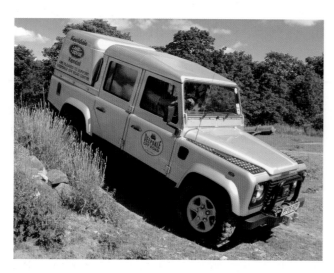

One of the most successful diversification enterprises is "Deepdale Off-Road". The course is designed to train participants in handling four-wheel-drive vehicles and trailers.

Graeme was conscious of the "Rambo" image of off-road driving, and began by underlining his genuine commitment to conducting an operation that would cause no damage to the environment, no disturbance of wildlife, and no inconvenience to neighbours. Consultation with the local council, the planning authorities, and the Farming and Wildlife Advisory Group were crucial. As a result he was given the "go-ahead". Deepdale Off-Road was born.

The fortunes of dairying continued to decline, and as his new venture prospered, there was only one way forward. The cows had to go so that Graeme could spend all his time and energy looking after his business, which has gone from strength to strength.

My friends, the dales farmers, may have had a pretty raw deal from the world's politicians and economists in recent years. They, like young Arthur, have learned how unfair life can be. But they'll survive thanks to the strength of character, adaptability, and tenacity that has been bred into them to survive in these hills over the centuries.

I wish them well.

37 By Hook or by Crook

Imagine, if you will, a typical March day in the Pennine hills. Sleet is flying in a stiff Pennine breeze. It isn't coming down vertically, it's travelling horizontally. Each pellet of frozen rain stings and pits the exposed face of anyone who turns into the wind.

Add to this scenario a young veterinary student who is earning a few pounds and a lot of experience working for a month as an assistant shepherd during the frantic activity of lambing time. A lamb has become separated from its mother. Its plaintive little bleating noises underline its distress. A few hours with an empty stomach in these conditions will mean certain doom for the little creature.

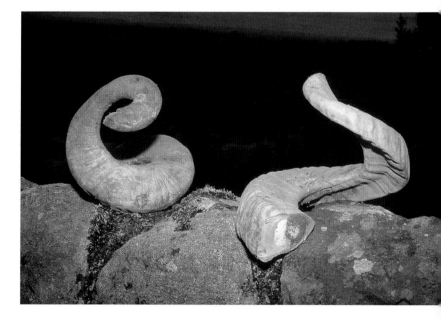

The raw materials.

Ignoring the biting sleet, wellies slipping on the winter-sodden turf, the young veterinary student is in hot pursuit of the little fellow. He nears his quarry. He gently crooks the handle of his stick around the breast of the lamb and the race is over. He reels in the prodigal, tucks it under his arm, and trudges off to reunite mother and child.

The young veterinary student was, of course, me. I learned so much in that month under my mentor, Bill Tweddle, at High House Farm, not least of which was the adept use of the shepherd's crook.

The shepherd's crook is such a basic tool. Its simplest function is that of a walking stick to steady the owner as he crosses the uneven ground of the moors. Another function is its use in catching sheep. By gently placing the head of the stick around the neck of an adult sheep or, as above, around the breast of a small lamb, the shepherd can restrain the animal. Its third use is as a probe, when searching for sheep overblown by snow. And fourthly it can be used as an extension of the arm to guide sheep through a gateway. You'll see this at the "penning" stage at a sheepdog trial.

A fifth use was related to me by a client who lived on what was probably the most remote farm in the practice. It was, literally, miles from his nearest neighbour. One night, returning home across the desolate moor, he was caught in a sudden blizzard. When his car foundered, he set off to continue his journey on foot, but as the powdery flakes swirled about him he lost his bearings completely.

He realised the danger of wandering off in an aimless direction in a "white-out" on the treacherous fell. He could have easily become trapped in steep-sided clefts in the peat or in one of the many bogs. However, he also realised that he had to keep moving, so he planted his crook in the snow and walked around it all night. At first light he regained his bearings and managed to complete his journey home. His crook and his quick thinking had saved his life.

The making of a horn-handled stick is a long process requiring much patience. In the Pennines the favoured material for the handle is the horn from an aged Swaledale tup. This must be boiled before being squeezed between two metal plates to straighten the curve. Then comes the carving and finishing. At the height of the BSE epidemic, it was ruled that all sheep heads from abattoirs must be incinerated. The stick-dressers, at a stroke, lost their source of raw material. Fortunately the rule was abandoned a few years later.

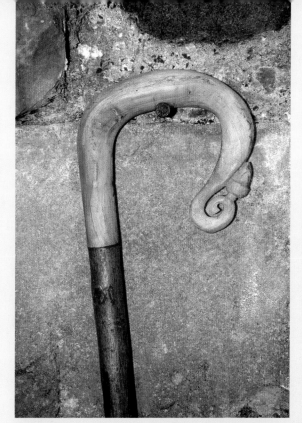

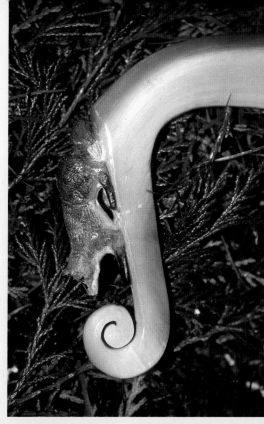

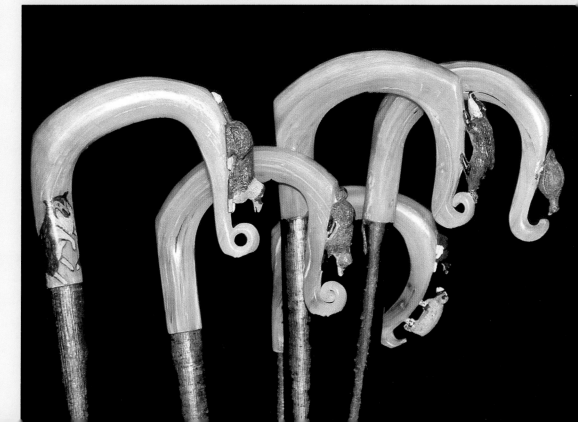

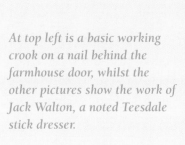

At top left is a basic working crook on a nail behind the farmhouse door, whilst the other pictures show the work of Jack Walton, a noted Teesdale stick dresser.

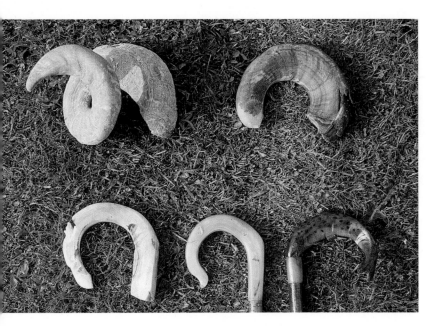

Some of the stages in making a stick.

The shank can be of ash, holly, hazel, or fruitwoods, although hazel is probably the commonest. The stick-maker will tie these in bundles and leave them to season for at least a year. It is said that one noted stick-maker kept his for fifteen years before he would use them. In general it is better to cut shanks in the winter when there is less sap in the wood, although there is a school of thought that recommends cutting as soon as you see a suitable piece—"before anyone else sees it!"

Joining the shank and the handle is termed "marrying". This can be accomplished by boring into each and using dowel and glue to effect the joint.

Anyone who sees the array of intricately decorated sticks at country fairs and agricultural shows could be forgiven for imagining that stick-dressing is an ancient craft. Surprisingly this is not so. Until relatively recently the crook was a basic, no-frills tool with only the name of the maker or his farm scratched onto the stick and perhaps the sign of a thistle.

In 1933 George Snaith and Ned Henderson entered sticks at Thropton Show in Northumberland's Coquet valley. Each of these sticks had a handle in the shape of a trout. George and a group of friends eventually founded the Border Stick Dressers Association on 19 May 1951, although even then the only decoration seemed to be a thistle or a trout.

George passed on his skills to a young Northumbrian farmer, Norman Tulip, who became one of the greatest stick-dressers of all time.

Norman's sticks have been presented to most members of the Royal Family. Sadly Norman is no longer with us, but a collection of thirty-five of his sticks is on display in Alnwick Castle. One of Norman's sticks, which has a handle decorated with lobsters, took 450 hours to make.

Although I first learned to handle the shepherd's crook as a student, I never actually owned one until after I retired.

I was determined that my retirement would be a low-profile, no bally-hoo, no parties affair. I wanted to slip away quietly. However, one evening my wife, Chris, whisked me away to a hotel right at the top of the dale. A surprise party had been arranged by some of the farmers up there.

"Well, if I'm to get a present, I hope it's a horn-handled stick," I said to Chris.

It was. And to my delight it was made by Jack Walton of Newton Lodge, one of the finest stick-dressers in the dale.

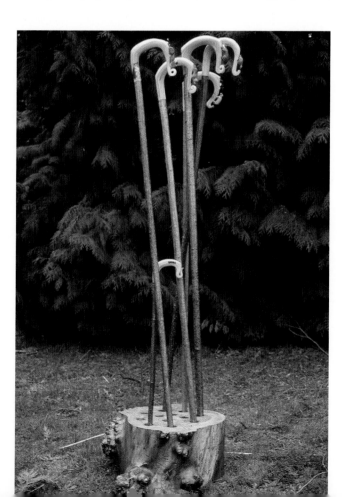

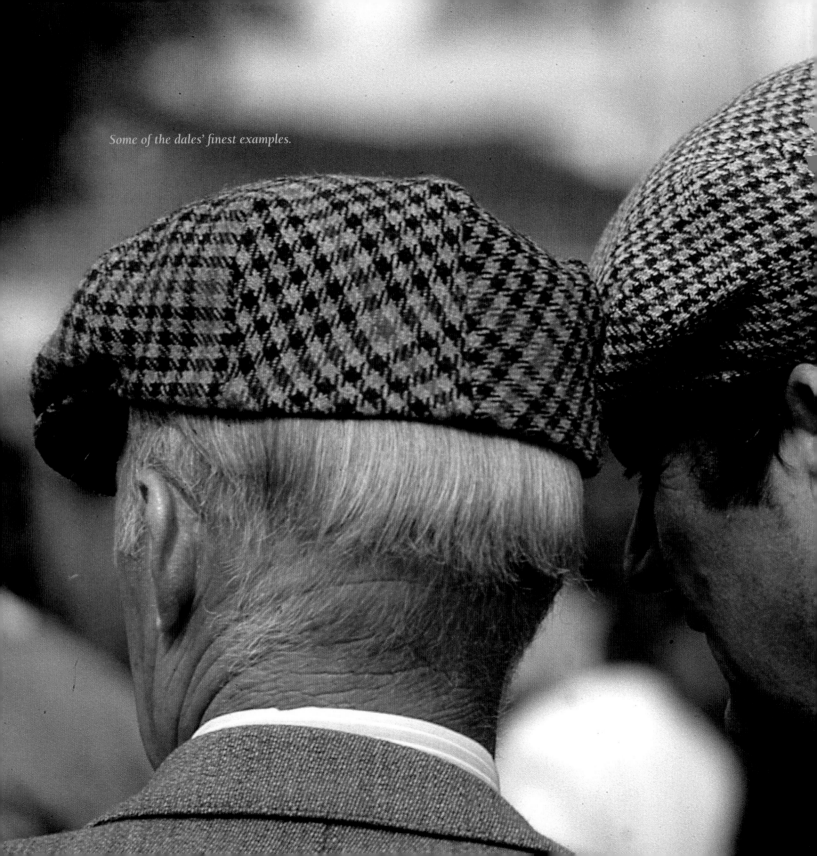

Some of the dales' finest examples.

38 Flat Hattery

I magine Royal Ascot without toppers, or Henley without boaters. Imagine guardsmen without bearskins, judges without horsehair wigs, high-ranking academics without mortarboards or university chancellors without huge, velvet, mediaeval caps.

Headgear may be functional, guarding a thinning pate from rain or sun, but hats are also a code of dress signifying something of the character or calling of the chap underneath.

In northern farming circles the crowning glory is the flat cap. Worn straight it might give a clue that the wearer is perhaps a bit formal. At a jaunty angle you can be sure that you can share a joke with this fellow. Whatever style, the older generation would always touch the peak of the cap when greeting a

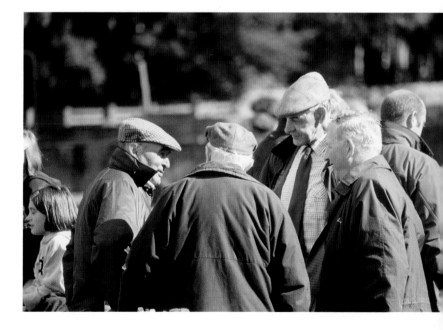

lady; a charming gesture which, sadly, is seldom seen nowadays.

On show day the Sunday-best model gets an airing, whilst the workday model with its rich patina of sump oil and cow muck hangs on a hook behind the farmhouse door.

There's a sure sign of the inveterate cap-bearer. When the farmer removes his cap, you may note a horizontal line across the upper forehead, above which is lilywhite skin that seldom sees the light of day. Below the line is the rest of the face, tanned to a ruddy hue by a lifetime of facing the elements.

Whether weighing up the livestock at the cattle mart, getting their hands dirty in the lambing pen, or wrestling with the spluttering engine of an ailing tractor, any self-respecting farmer would look naked if the ensemble weren't topped off by a downright sensible flat hat.

I've never been into headgear. Come to think of it, I can't think of many vets who were. But I can't think of many of my farming clients who weren't!

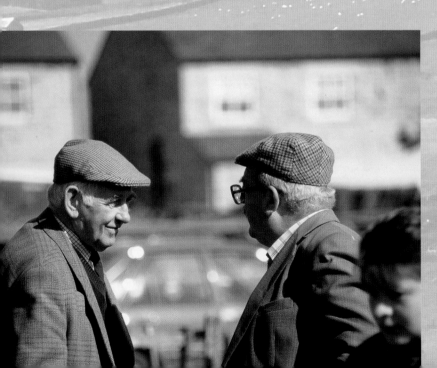

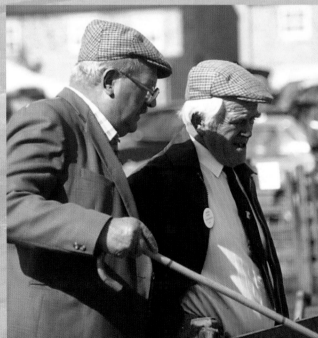

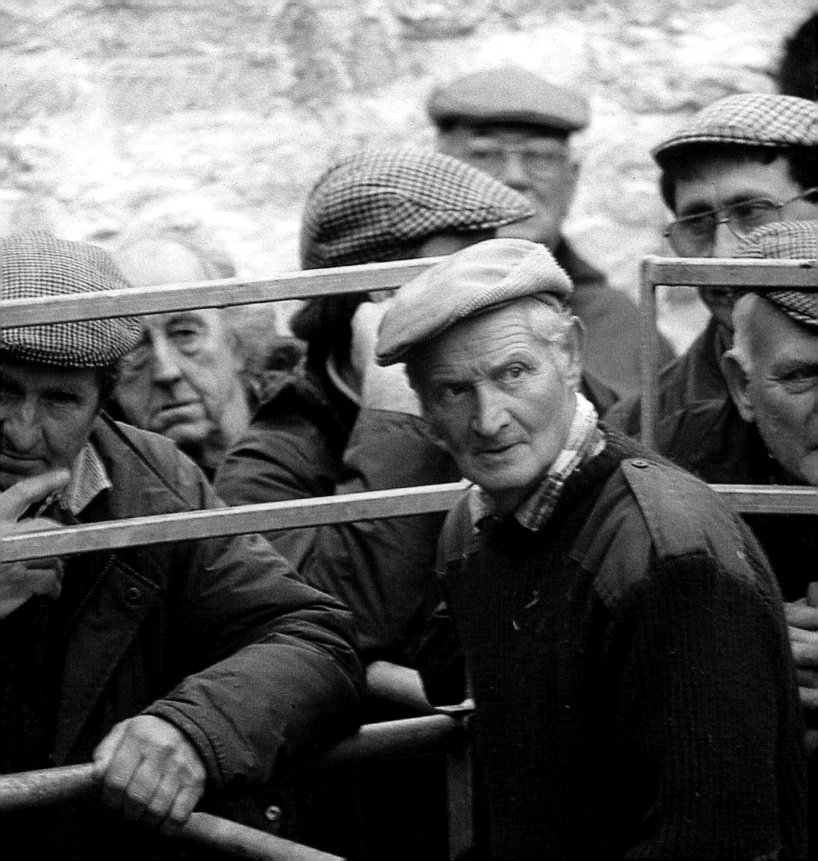

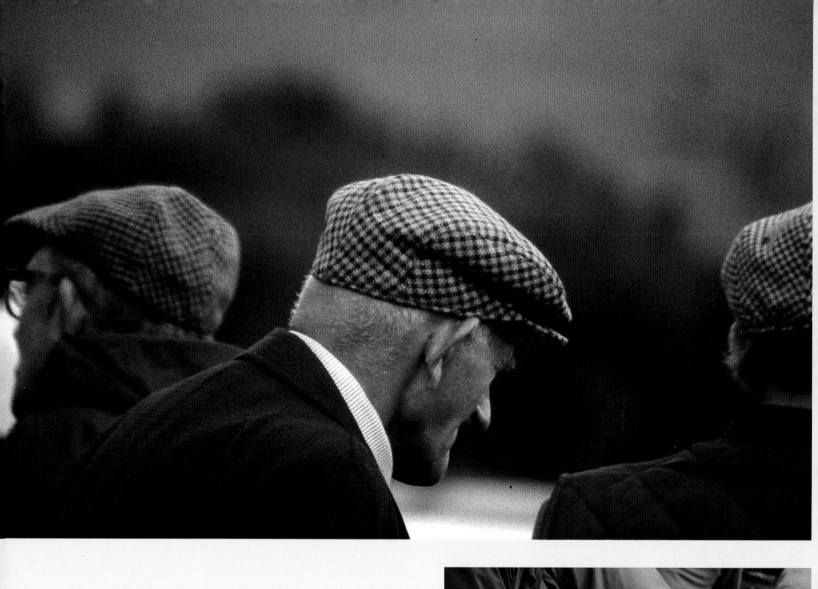
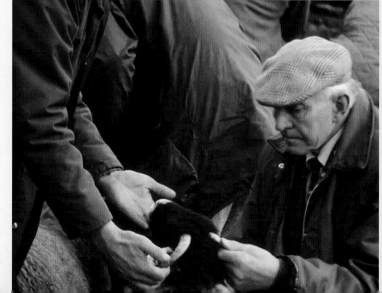

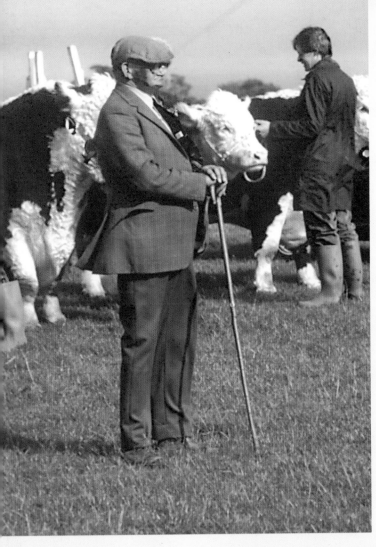

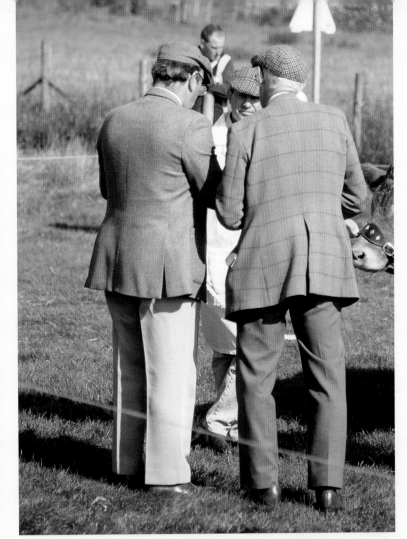

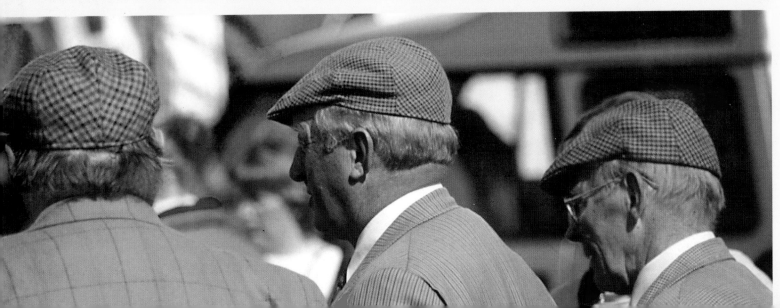